HARDING HOSPITAL
CLINICAL INTERNSHIP in ART THERAPY

THERAPEUTIC DANCE/MOVEMENT

Expressive Activities for Older Adults

Erna Caplow-Lindner M. S.

Leah Harpaz, M.A.

Sonya Samberg, G.D.T.

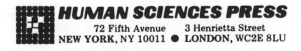

HUMAN SCIENCES PRESS

72 Fifth Avenue   3 Henrietta Street
NEW YORK, NY 10011 ● LONDON, WC2E 8LU

Printed in the United States of America
98765432

Library of Congress Cataloging in Publication Data

Caplow-Lindner, Erna
    Therapeutic dance/movement.

    Bibliography: p.
    Includes index.
    1. Aged – Rehabilitation. 2. Dance therapy.
3. Exercise for the aged. I. Harpaz, Leah,
joint author. II. Samberg, Sonya, joint author.
III. Title.
RC953.5.L56   615'.85   LC78-10931
ISBN 0-87705-340-5
ISBN 0-87705-347-2 pbk.

We dedicate this book
    to our husbands and families who have encouraged us
        and
    to the elderly who have taught us.

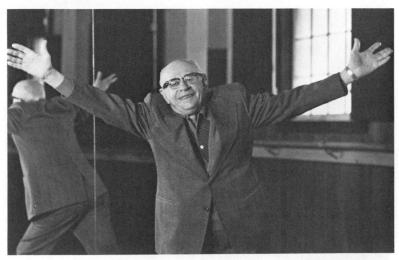

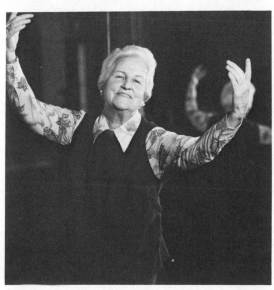

CONTENTS

NOTE TO THE SELF-HELP USER

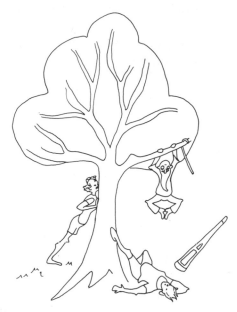

Although this book has been written to provide professionals with guidelines and specific material to conduct therapeutic movement sessions, the general reader will find its contents valuable for personal use.

The clearly explained exercises on pages 78–106 are arranged in separate groups of energetic, moderate and mild types. You can easily select the appropriate group of exercises to help you improve your flexibility, coordination, circulation, and muscle tone as you practice on your own or with a friend or two.

Chapter Four includes step by step techniques for conscious relaxation, correct breathing, and self-massage that can be followed independently by the non-professional adult.

If you have ever wanted hints on how to be more comfortable and safe while doing ordinary activities such as carrying, lifting, bathing, and getting in and out of cars, then you will welcome the detailed section on General Health Issues.

Each older adult who has been bothered by arthritis, poor sleeping habits, or digestive difficulties will discover practical suggestions and reassurances in Chapter Six.

And finally, try some of the dances and rhythm game ideas in Chapter Five to add joy and companionship to your life. You'll find the experience truly therapeutic!

Foreword

As a physician concerned with the health and care of aging people, I firmly support any activity that will motivate and cause older people to move and be more active physically and mentally, no matter what infirmity they may have. Movement, as this book points out, is the essence and secret of healthier and happier aging. Without it, the older person loses his ability to walk around and falls prey to the increasing doubts and hobgoblins of faltering old age. There is no question that proper exercise can improve physiologic and other musculoskeletal alterations in the elderly.

Therapeutic dance/movement, one of the more popular and growing ways to improve mobility and independence, offers a sound approach to the important problems of maintaining and improving mobility, balance, coordination, rhythm, endurance, strength and flexibility—all of which inevitably deteriorate with age but which exercise and activity can at least improve.

Therapeutic dance/movement combines the benefits of dancing, music, and socialization. Dance, a synthesizing art form, makes available to the aged the vital elements of rhythm, dramatic expression, spatial design and physical dynamics which too long have been limited to the young. Dance therapy, utilizing rhythm and movement for self expression and communication, penetrates to the core of human experience and expression and aids in the healthy integration of mind and body.

Music, the second major element in therapeutic dance/movement program, is a powerful mood modifier useful therapeutically to calm, soothe, stimulate and to rebuild a more healthful emotional pattern for participants.

Together with the group work aspects, therapeutic dance/movement helps older people to develop more outlets for positive and negative emotions, social interactions, physical activity and relaxation and assists them to establish a more meaningful relationship with others. The expressive, creative activity of therapeutic dance/movement is an excellent way to develop a greater sense of personal identity, wider resources and awareness of community relations. Obviously, "in dancing with you, I accept you!"

Such programs call into play nonverbal communication as an integral element of therapy, stimulate greater sensory awareness and establish new neural patterns. For the aged with deterioration of the central nervous system and impairment of sensory perception, it may be far more helpful and reassuring for them to touch, feel and move in therapeutic dance/movement than to listen, hear and think in a more intellectual approach.

To be sure, these benefits of therapeutic dance/movement vary according to the ability, personality and devotion of the dance therapist. This book offers students and qualified professionals who seek careers as dance therapists the necessary information concerning programming. Included in this text are music, exercises and the equally essential information and insights necessary to work successfully with older people.

Although therapeutic dance/movement appears useful for people of all ages, it requires further documentation and research, as the authors recognize. They stress the importance of keeping adequate records that will justify the existence, support and expense of therapeutic dance/-movement programs for older people. Of interest are their results which suggest slight to moderate improvement mainly in the torso and upper limbs of geriatric patients. Lower limb mobility and space orientation improve less dramatically through therapeutic dance programs in this age group. These results may be related to the large numbers of non-ambulatory clients in this sampling.

Therapeutic dance/movement is a new marshalling of movement and dance therapeutically. My own experience with such exercise for older people indicates to me its value. I suppose I am more than slightly influenced by a memory of several years ago when I watched the legendary Ruth St. Denis, then in her late 80's, at a performance honoring Ted Shawn at Jacob's Pillow in the Berkshire Mountains. Off stage, Ruth St. Denis walked stiffly and slowly due to musculoskeletal and other age-associated impairments. On stage, her joints and muscles loosened, her years dropped away as she instinctively glided and pirouetted across the stage like the great dancer she had been years before.

Recently, I had the good fortune to be in charge of a conference on exercise for older people where the authors of this book played their music and demonstrated their techniques. Like other professionals at the program, I soon found myself keeping time with the music and then joining the therapeutic dance/movement demonstration. I agree with the distinguished physiatrist at my side who commented, "You know, this is undoubtedly the best way for older people to exercise for greater mobility, strength, happiness and independence."

Read this book yourself and see if you don't agree.

Raymond Harris, M.D.
President, Center for the Study of Aging
Clinical Associate Professor
of Medicine, Albany Medical College
Albany, New York

AUTHORS' PREFACE

This book is the result of an interrelationship among three colleagues with uniquely different backgrounds and talents in the fields of dance, movement education, and group work. Each of us has had extensive training and experience in the use of rhythmic movement with the older adult and we have each enjoyed careers as dancers. Over the last 10 years we have successfully been working with the aged in nursing facilities, old age homes, and senior citizen centers. Our programs have been offered to the blind, severely handicapped, and the energetic, well elderly.

Recently we combined our talents to produce a musical recording with rhythmic activity instructions for special populations. And in the past few years we have presented numerous training workshops and demonstrations for the staffs of geriatric facilities. The participants and staff of the various agencies where we have conducted these programs have expressed an overwhelming need for a leader's guide to therapeutic movement sessions for the aging. Movement therapy has only been recognized professionally for ap- proximately 20 years and the significance of geriatric dance therapy has just been acknowledged within the last few years. Thus, many professionals in the field of geriatrics have not received training in dance/movement and are eager to become competent in its use.

We believe in encouraging people to use their bodies to the fullest extent as instruments of communication within a social context. Because our viewpoint emphasizes the creative impulses in everyone, teachers and therapists with almost any age group will be able to adapt our mate- rial.

Recently within the health-related professions, it has become less important to separate therapeutic modalities. Dancers and expressive arts therapists have found that ap- proaches that utilize music, movement, and communica- tion skills all overlap. Therefore, this book is addressed to all the people who are interested in working with the disori- ented, the disabled, the isolated, and the individual with limited capabilities. For example, there are activity sugges- tions that may help nurses and gerontologists who are con- cerned with the apathy and withdrawal that is often found during long-term confinement or chronic illness. Social workers and psychiatric staff workers may appreciate the use of dance/movement therapy as a stimulus for talking about problems and as an aid to socialization. The physical therapist and geriatric aides may see possibilities for using rhythmic elements to improve performance, proprioceptor response, and the consistency of activity. And many aspects of the dance program may appeal to the occupational ther- apist and the activities specialists as constructive group recreation.

We know that since all the arts are personal expres- sions, there will be many different ways of working with dance movement for the elderly. Our approach is unique in that, in addition to offering exercises adapted to the limitations of balance, coordination, and strength, it includes variations of creative dance, yoga, and folk dance. The knowledge gained from years spent teaching creative dance to children and adults and from performing and choreographing has contributed to the material we draw on for our geriatric groups.

In this book we have written about the four segments of the elderly spectrum: the well aged, the physically limited, the severely handicapped, and the withdrawn or regressed. In order to show the fullest scope of therapeutic benefit that movement sessions can offer the aging, we have presented activities to encourage socialization, self-expression, positive mental recall, improved body image, and sensory stimulation that can be used in geriatric situations. We try to reach out to the whole person. So many times the older adult, especially the institutionalized person, is treated in a fragmented way. We have found that our movement skills can enrich the lives of others and bring us great rewards. It has been possible for us to maintain the capabilities of many aging individuals. We have also been able to revive dormant skills and share in new experiences with our geriatric groups.

We hope that the respect and the faith we have in the dignity of each person will be evident. We do not view our program merely as exercise sessions or isolated activity but as a projection and an extension of each individual's total life experience. Therefore, our purposes in writing this book will be fulfilled if we inspire recognition of the need for improved therapeutic movement programs for the aged and if we influence further creative efforts in that direction.

Erna Caplow Lindner, M.S., Movement Therapist
Associate Professor of Health, Physical Education and
 Recreation
Nassau Community College
Garden City, New York

Leah Harpaz, M.A., Movement Therapist
Executive Vice President for Dance
North Shore Community Arts Center
Great Neck, New York

Sonya Samberg, G.D.T., Movement Therapist
Geriatric Movement Specialist
Frederic D. Zeman Center for Instruction at the Jewish
   Home and Hospital for Aged,
   New York, New York

ACKNOWLEDGMENTS

WE ARE INDEBTED TO

    our predecessors and colleagues who have inspired us by their contributions to dance and movement for the aging.

    our friends Bernard Kassoy, Alma Rosenthal, Peter Ruchman, Robert Blucher, and Benjamin Scherman for generously sharing their artistic talents with us so that this book could be illustrated with their original drawings and photographs.

    our mentors, Norma Fox, Editor-in-Chief, Human Sciences Press and Maureen Conway, Project Editor, Cobb/Dunlop Publisher Services, who made the transitions from idea to manuscript to book possible by their patience, encouragement, and salient advice.

WE OWE THANKS TO

    the following administrators and geriatric specialists for their practical assistance and support of our work:

Zenon Arribalzago, formerly Director, Highbridge Senior Citizen Center, Bronx, N.Y.; Mary Feldman, Group Social Worker, Vacations and Community Services for the Blind, New York City; Paula Gross Gray, Director of Activities, and Anna Evansoff Viruet, Supervisor of Activities, Jewish Home and Hospital for the Aged, New York City; Edith Shapiro, Director of Activities, Roberta Salshutz, Activities Therapist, Frances Komarin, Social Worker, Frances Nissenbaum, Social Worker, and Claire Kaminsky, Head Nurse, Jewish Institute for Geriatric Care, New Hyde Park, N.Y.; Celia Lickver, Supervisor of Senior Citizen Programs, Samuel Field YM-YWHA, Little Neck, N.Y.; Sister Annunciato, Director, Bedford Park Senior Citizen Center at St. Philip Neri Church, Bronx, N.Y.; Ronald Szezypkowski, formerly Director, Education for Aging Center, Continuing Education Department, Bronx Community College, Bronx, N.Y.; Carolyn Du Sablon, Chief of Therapeutic Recreation, Anne Cash, Recreation Therapist, and Arnold Feinman, Recreation Therapist, Rehabilitation Division of Peninsula Hospital, Far Rockaway, N.Y.; Ben Zion Altman, Director, Rabbi Mordecai Waxman, Spiritual Leader, and Rabbi Carl Wolkin, Advisor of the Senior Mitsva Group, Temple Israel, Great Neck, N.Y.

the following persons and agencies for their cooperation with our efforts to assemble the training workshops and research that contributed to this book:

Sara Yurman, Registrar, Zeman Institute for Instruction of the Jewish Home and Hospital for the Aged, New York City; Janice Josephson, Director of Community Services, and Dr. Sanda Costescu, former Medical Staff Member, Jewish Institute for Geriatric Care, New Hyde Park, N.Y.; Sigmund C. Taft, formerly Director of Activities, Jewish Home and Hospital for the Aged, New York City; Ethel Paley, Executive Director, Friends and Relatives of the Institutionalized Aged, New York City; Elizabeth Zubow, Director of Activities; A. Holly Patterson Nursing Home, Uniondale, N.Y.; the Library Staffs of the Manhattan Veterans Administration Hospital, New York City; Nassau Community College, Garden City, N.Y.; and the Public Library of Great Neck, N.Y.

Chapter 1

THEORETICAL CONSIDERATIONS

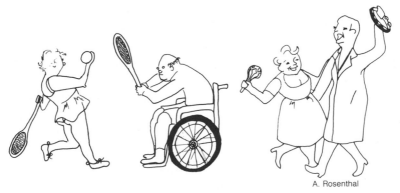

A. Rosenthal

SOCIOLOGICAL IMPLICATIONS OF AGING

Attitudes of Society Toward the Aged

The attitude of society toward its elderly has varied throughout history. Some cultures adopted a protective and respectful attitude toward their older members, while among many primitive people it was the custom to abandon the elderly and to let them die. The Chinese honored and held the aged in such high esteem that they developed a system of ancestor worship. An example of the insecure and highly competitive situation in which the elderly are considered a burden on the state is that of the Nazis who disposed of their aged and infirm. From various studies we can see that societies, which have attained high cultural and economic levels and a stable family structure, nurture and revere their older members. And yet the recent emergence of the nuclear family concept, which emphasizes generational independence, has prompted the isolation of the aging parent, grandparent, and other old relatives in some areas of our affluent society. This, together with the work ethic and money values in our culture, contribute to the decreased worth of the retired, financially restricted older American.

Position of the Aged in the United States

The history of our country has shown that until recently our government did not assume any responsibility toward its senior members. The destitute elderly could only get help from the limited local facilities such as almshouses, jails, or insane asylums. It was in 1935, with the introduction of Social Security, that the national government took the first major step to improve the economic life of its senior citizens. In 1950 President Harry Truman urged that the First National Conference on Aging be held. This conference developed guidelines for action and set up agencies to take care of the needs and problems of the elderly. The Second Conference on Aging was held in 1961 and again focused on the problems and potentials of older Americans. In 1965 the Older Americans Act was passed, establishing the U.S. Administration on Aging in the Department of Health, Education and Welfare. This act also provided Medicare for the aged to help finance medical needs. Included in the legislation was encouragement for the "pursuit of meaningful activity for the elderly within the widest range of civic, cultural, and recreational opportunities." The Third National Conference on Aging, held in 1971, recommended that Home Care Service be provided so that elderly persons could maintain their own homes as long as possible. It stated that "every person has a right to achieve a sense of spiritual well being" and that one of the long-range goals is "to prepare every citizen for retirement 'to' something rather than 'from' something by providing him with outlets for creative expression." Thus it becomes apparent that in the past 40 years, there has developed an awareness and a desire on the part of many Americans for action and programs that would help senior citizens to solve their problems and to realize their potentials more fully. The federal government now supports many programs that serve the special needs of the aged in their own local communities.

Recent Developments Concerning the Elderly

The intensified activity in the field of programming for the aged has been partially spurred on by recent developments such as (1) the nursing home investigations in New York State, 1975–1976, (2) the reports of the Moreland Act Commission, (3) the growing force of consumerism in general, and (4) the change of the mandatory retirement age in many fields of employment from 65 to 70 years of age. The elderly, particularly, are becoming organized in self-advocacy programs through groups such as The League of Women Voters, The Grey Panthers, and FRIA (Friends and Relatives of the Institutionalized Aged). Another, and extremely important, factor is the enormous increase in the number of people over the age of 65 in our society today. All of these influences have contributed to the realization that one measure of our society will be the quality of life of our older people. We now evaluate the total health of the elderly, not only by the absence of physical disease, but by their state of mind and their place in the social structure.

Population Statistics of the Elderly

In 1900 there were only three million elderly people in the United States, or 4% of the total population. Now there are over 21 million, 10% of the total. Projections for the year 2000 place our aged population at about 29 million (1). This increase is due partly to the rise in the birthrate from the late 1800s through the early 1920s. Two other important factors were the tremendous number of immigrants who came to the United States before World War I and the increased life span brought about by medical progress in curing serious disease plus the improved physical fitness and nutrition programs.

While the proportion of the elderly in the total population has risen, there has also been an increase in the average age of that group. The percentage of the aged from 65 to 69 years old has been decreasing, while that of 75 years old and older has increased. In 1900 the proportion of those who were 75 and over was 29% of the aged; by 1970 this proportion had climbed to 38%.

At present, a large number of the elderly are female. In 1930 the numbers of men and women were about equal. In 1970 there were 11.6 million elderly women and 8.4 million elderly men. A white male in today's society can look forward to a life expectancy of 72 years and his female counterpart to one of 82 years.

Economic Status of the Aged

In 1973 the income level of 16% of the population over 65 was below the poverty level (2). It is therefore difficult for the elderly to obtain health care, especially prevention-oriented services. It limits their ability to maintain a well-balanced diet and provide suitable clothing and comfortable living conditions that would be conducive to well-being and a healthy self-image.

Mental Health of the Aged

Because of the foregoing economic and social factors, the mental health problems are particularly severe in the aged

Wheels," in which volunteers deliver food to those aged who can not prepare their own meals. Another very important program is "Early Alert." If the letter carrier notices an accumulation of mail in the mailboxes of the elderly person enrolled in this program, he or she contacts the appropriate authorities who can enter the apartment or house and give aid if needed.

Peer groups also offer assistance through such programs as: "Knock for Your Neighbor," in which neighbors knock on each others' doors daily to check up on each other; "Sunshine" programs of regular visitations and "Hotline for the Aged," a telephone calling arrangement for consistent contacts.

Services for the Institutionalized Aged

Because of the severely restricted capabilities of the residents and the confining nature of a nursing facility, special recreational and adjunctive services must be provided for the institutionalized person. Rehabilitative and maintenance programs such as physical and occupational therapies and music, dance/movement, and art activities are becoming integral parts of the care of the confined elderly. The focus for the aged is on doing and being a contributing participant rather than a passive recipient.

Future Training Needs

The newly established disciplines of gerontology and geriatrics are growing rapidly to keep pace with the enormous increase in the proportion of elderly in our population. A survey has shown that 1275 schools offer at least one course in gerontology and the outlook is for continued government aid for training programs. The demand for professionals in the field will accelerate over the next 10 years with estimates of 1000 additional psychiatrists, 2000

population. In addition to the economic and demographic facts pointing to difficulties for the elderly in our country, there are also the cultural pressures that force inactivity, dependency, and even virtual exile on our senior citizens. Dr. James Birren, director of the Ethel Percy Andrus Gerontology Center of the University of Southern California has said, ". . . it's not bad to be old; it's bad to be unhealthy; it's bad to be lonely . . ." (3). Without strong personal resources or outside assistance, a constructive mental outlook is extremely difficult to achieve. That may be why we find that 30% of the residents in public mental hospitals are 65 years old and over.

We need to publicize and offer support to the obvious fact that the older adult can be productive and creative well into his/her eighth and ninth decade of life. Senility and uselessness are not the absolute destiny of the aging as we see by the lives of Martha Graham, Pablo Picasso, Georgia O'Keeffe, George Bernard Shaw, Leonardo da Vinci, Arturo Toscanini, Bernard Baruch, and countless others.

Until fairly recently, the potential for change and rehabilitation for the aged was considered too limited or nonexistent. The adage, "You can't teach an old dog new tricks" seems to have been repudiated by numerous studies of the mental and physical capabilities of people throughout their life span. There are now myriad examples of people whose lives have been renewed and enriched at relatively advanced ages. The contemporary trends of opening doors for new educational opportunities and career changes for the older adult indicate this recent societal interest.

Even the use of psychotherapy is now recommended for the elderly. Dr. Ernest Kovacs, a psychiatrist who works with older adults at the psychiatric division of the Long Island Jewish-Hillside Medical Center in New York, finds that psychotherapy and counseling are effective for short-term goals with people 60 and 70 and older. They are able to talk of their feelings of isolation, their physical problems,

and their family relationships. Through group and professional help they are able to work through negative attitudes
and change undesired behavior patterns so that they can
lead more productive and enjoyable lives (4).

Dr. Brice Pitt, a recognized authority in English gerontology circles, is essentially optimistic about the prospects
of eventual recovery for innumerable elderly persons, with
improved care and understanding. He says that what is
needed is " . . . social measures which enable an old person
to live as full and independent a life as possible, and the
principles and techniques by which a patient is assisted to
make the most of his residual abilities" (5).

Elderly Life-Style Options

Today the diversity of living patterns available to the elderly presents challenges to the public and private sectors
for providing services to the aging.

Between 1960 and 1970 the family status of the elderly
changed. A growing proportion of them are now maintaining independent households rather than living with relatives or residing in institutions. In 1960 only 25% of older
women were living alone; but in 1970 33% were in this
category. Relatively few of the elderly in the United States
live in homes for the aged. The proportions are 3% for
men and 4% for women as of 1970 (6). Of these nursing
home residents, the majority, 63%, were ambulatory, 20%
spent part of the day in a wheelchair, 11% were confined
to a chair or wheelchair all day, and 6% were restricted to
total bed rest (7).

The past decade has been characterized by the proliferation of age-segregated communities such as "Leisure
World" in California and "Leisure Village" on Long Island. Here senior citizens can have privacy, protection, and
recreational activities within a few steps of their homes.
Some prefer to live in "golden age" apartment hotels with

communal dining and maid services. Another kind of
arrangement is the apartment residence with cooper
owned or rented units where planned activities are o
These are either privately or philanthropically funde
amples are "Springvale" in Westchester County
York, and "Century Village" in West Palm Beach, F
Many unions and large business organizations have
lished retirement homes or housing for their me
The retired person may be able to live more econo
with companionship and often with many perso
social services. There are also apartment residenc
ated with nursing homes and hospitals where skil
is provided. Typical of this type in New York State
"Isabella Apartments" in Manhattan and the
House" in the Bronx. A recent development has
retirement communities of trailer camps, privatel
organized by governmental agencies such as Hou
Urban Development (HUD). And now, communal
ments among groups of friends, newly retired,
sulted in joint buying, building, and maintainir
residences in Pennsylvania, Connecticut, Virg
other areas.

Services for the Independent Aged

The benefits for senior citizens who live at home
nized by authorities as twofold: for the aged,
living is more self-fulfilling and humanistic; fo
is less costly to provide home care services. G
funding is provided to support such important
day care centers, senior citizen groups, golden
and outpatient centers for both recreational a
services. The elderly who live in their own ho
essential services through community outreac
that provide part-time homemakers, visiting
social workers. Another community service i

clinical psychologists, 4000 psychiatric social workers, and 10,000 other specialists, in addition to medically trained staff members, required to provide services for the aged (8).

Because of the intent of Titles III and VII of the Older Americans Act and Title XX of the Social Security Act, there has been a general upgrading of program offerings and improved staff training in all publicly supported and licensed geriatric facilities. The American Hospital Association noted at their conference in 1971, "Winds of Change," that " . . . medicare . . . is recommending that extended care facilities provide the appropriate diversional programs directed by a qualified staff member." This indicates a " . . . long-overdue recognition of the fact that activities should be part of the health care plan and that they have value just as nursing, physical therapy, dietary, and all other services do" (9).

BACKGROUND OF THERAPEUTIC MOVEMENT FOR GERIATRICS

Historical Development of Therapeutic Dance

The roots of dance therapy may be found in ancient times in the tribal rituals of almost every pretechnological society. Primitive peoples have always sought physical means to communicate with the supernatural and to heal their spiritual ills. Rhythmic and symbolic movement has provided expression for people's fears and joys throughout the centuries.

Dance therapy, as we know it today, is a relatively new field that began about 30 years ago at the end of World War II. At that time, because of the extensive use of drugs for mental and emotional illness, it was necessary to find nonverbal therapeutic methods to reach the mentally ill patients. Two pioneers who utilized the improvisational self-expression processes of modern dance as an adjunct to psychotherapy at that time, were Marion Chace of Washington, D.C., and Blanche Evan of New York City. Their work, in very different settings and from uniquely personal viewpoints, provided therapeutic experiences involving group interaction, individual expression, and heightened body awareness for the participants.

From that beginning, dance therapy has developed into a tool for defining and directing individual progress toward well-being (sense of comfort, adjustment, and fulfillment) and has become an independent form of non-verbal therapy.

The American Dance Therapy Association was established in 1964 with Marion Chace as its first president. Since that time the profession has worked to establish standards for training and practice that include certification or "registry" for clinical therapists and has encouraged scholarship and research through journals and regular national and international conferences. The development of academic programs for undergraduate and graduate level college degrees in dance therapy is a fairly recent indication that the field is being recognized and accepted by colleagues in the "helping" professions.

At this time, action at the governmental level is taking place to promote the necessary funding and administrative organization for jobs and programming in dance therapy. Individual leaders in the field are making their work and their needs known to the public. The other creative arts therapies, art, music, and drama, together with dance, have joined forces to bring their message to Washington and the state capitals.

It is now acknowledged that dance therapy is effective in the treatment and conduct of programs for individuals with a wide range of physical and mental problems. Emotionally disturbed children and adults, institutionalized psychiatric patients, the physically handicapped, the elderly, and the learning disabled have all benefited from the use of dance/movement therapy. Therefore, in the 1970s dance therapy has achieved an equal status with the other health related professions.

Definition of Dance Therapy

Dance therapy is the use of rhythmic movement as a means of self-expression and communication that aids in the healthy integration of mind and body. The motivation to treat or improve the well-being of the participants is essential to the therapeutic character of the activity.

The concepts of modern dance, which utilizes movement improvisation with its relationship to time, space, and energy, laid the groundwork for the therapeutic use of dance. Dance therapy applies the interrelationships of movement elements, such as the amount of energy, type of flow, pace of action, and use of space to gain insight into the personality of the individual and to provide outlets for expression and socialization.

Special Needs of the Aging for Dance Therapy

Because the aging process is characterized by the onset of physical limitations and emotional stresses, it is vital to find outlets for self-expression and opportunities for social interaction, physical activity, and relaxation techniques. "The buildup of tension in the elderly can produce such symptoms as insomnia, fretfulness, and restlessness. The elderly often turn inward upon themselves their unrealised aggressive tendencies. These become a self-destructive force, leading to depression, which in turn, may increase tendencies toward psychosomatic diseases or lead to sudden outbursts of rage" (10). In addition, the normal process of disengagement, which takes place as one ages, is often accompanied by abnormal responses of withdrawal

and depression that may be ameliorated through movement activity and the leader's guidance.

Dr. Paul Schilder, an English authority on body image
and ego development, notes that "Movement is a great
uniting factor between the different parts of one's own
body" (11). He emphasizes the benefits of sensation and
perception through which a person becomes aware of
his/her relationship to the outside surroundings. Opportunities for movement provide experiences through which an
individual can build a more accurate body image.

Geriatric movement sessions help participants to discover pleasure in moving and through that, to find pleasure
in living. According to J. B. Helm and K. L. Gill, " . . . such
programs (dance therapy), if effectively supported, can
have a significant effect in reducing the resident population
of our mental institutions, as well as improving the quality
of life for our elderly" (12).

Purposes of Therapeutic Movement Sessions for the Elderly

Therapeutic movement sessions are ideally offered to discover, prevent, arrest, and reverse the damaging effects of
aging. Opportunities to express emotions, both positive
and negative, and to release tensions through movement
experiences are invaluable parts of the therapeutic session.
The movement therapist also offers stimulation for constructive recall, reality contacts, and social interaction. We
are working to promote a freer relationship between body
and mind by encouraging affirmative and meaningful gestures and movement.

The physical activity of the program produces the development of improved body alignment, increased range of
motion, and relaxation for the reduction of stress. If we
increase the range of movement and give opportunities for
more physical experience, we are helping to increase the

population. In addition to the economic and demographic facts pointing to difficulties for the elderly in our country, there are also the cultural pressures that force inactivity, dependency, and even virtual exile on our senior citizens. Dr. James Birren, director of the Ethel Percy Andrus Gerontology Center of the University of Southern California has said, ". . . it's not bad to be old; it's bad to be unhealthy; it's bad to be lonely . . ." (3). Without strong personal resources or outside assistance, a constructive mental outlook is extremely difficult to achieve. That may be why we find that 30% of the residents in public mental hospitals are 65 years old and over.

We need to publicize and offer support to the obvious fact that the older adult can be productive and creative well into his/her eighth and ninth decade of life. Senility and uselessness are not the absolute destiny of the aging as we see by the lives of Martha Graham, Pablo Picasso, Georgia O'Keeffe, George Bernard Shaw, Leonardo da Vinci, Arturo Toscanini, Bernard Baruch, and countless others.

Until fairly recently, the potential for change and rehabilitation for the aged was considered too limited or nonexistent. The adage, "You can't teach an old dog new tricks" seems to have been repudiated by numerous studies of the mental and physical capabilities of people throughout their life span. There are now myriad examples of people whose lives have been renewed and enriched at relatively advanced ages. The contemporary trends of opening doors for new educational opportunities and career changes for the older adult indicate this recent societal interest.

Even the use of psychotherapy is now recommended for the elderly. Dr. Ernest Kovacs, a psychiatrist who works with older adults at the psychiatric division of the Long Island Jewish-Hillside Medical Center in New York, finds that psychotherapy and counseling are effective for short-term goals with people 60 and 70 and older. They are able to talk of their feelings of isolation, their physical problems, and their family relationships. Through group and professional help they are able to work through negative attitudes and change undesired behavior patterns so that they can lead more productive and enjoyable lives (4).

Dr. Brice Pitt, a recognized authority in English gerontology circles, is essentially optimistic about the prospects of eventual recovery for innumerable elderly persons, with improved care and understanding. He says that what is needed is " . . . social measures which enable an old person to live as full and independent a life as possible, and the principles and techniques by which a patient is assisted to make the most of his residual abilities" (5).

Elderly Life-Style Options

Today the diversity of living patterns available to the elderly presents challenges to the public and private sectors for providing services to the aging.

Between 1960 and 1970 the family status of the elderly changed. A growing proportion of them are now maintaining independent households rather than living with relatives or residing in institutions. In 1960 only 25% of older women were living alone; but in 1970 33% were in this category. Relatively few of the elderly in the United States live in homes for the aged. The proportions are 3% for men and 4% for women as of 1970 (6). Of these nursing home residents, the majority, 63%, were ambulatory, 20% spent part of the day in a wheelchair, 11% were confined to a chair or wheelchair all day, and 6% were restricted to total bed rest (7).

The past decade has been characterized by the proliferation of age-segregated communities such as "Leisure World" in California and "Leisure Village" on Long Island. Here senior citizens can have privacy, protection, and recreational activities within a few steps of their homes. Some prefer to live in "golden age" apartment hotels with communal dining and maid services. Another kind of living arrangement is the apartment residence with cooperatively owned or rented units where planned activities are offered. These are either privately or philanthropically funded. Examples are "Springvale" in Westchester County, New York, and "Century Village" in West Palm Beach, Florida. Many unions and large business organizations have established retirement homes or housing for their members. The retired person may be able to live more economically, with companionship and often with many personal and social services. There are also apartment residences affiliated with nursing homes and hospitals where skilled care is provided. Typical of this type in New York State are the "Isabella Apartments" in Manhattan and the "Kittay House" in the Bronx. A recent development has been the retirement communities of trailer camps, privately built or organized by governmental agencies such as Housing and Urban Development (HUD). And now, communal arrangements among groups of friends, newly retired, have resulted in joint buying, building, and maintaining shared residences in Pennsylvania, Connecticut, Virginia, and other areas.

Services for the Independent Aged

The benefits for senior citizens who live at home are recognized by authorities as twofold: for the aged, this way of living is more self-fulfilling and humanistic; for society, it is less costly to provide home care services. Government funding is provided to support such important facilities as day care centers, senior citizen groups, golden age clubs, and outpatient centers for both recreational and medical services. The elderly who live in their own homes receive essential services through community outreach programs that provide part-time homemakers, visiting nurses, and social workers. Another community service is "Meals on

Wheels," in which volunteers deliver food to those aged who can not prepare their own meals. Another very important program is "Early Alert." If the letter carrier notices an accumulation of mail in the mailboxes of the elderly person enrolled in this program, he or she contacts the appropriate authorities who can enter the apartment or house and give aid if needed.

Peer groups also offer assistance through such programs as: "Knock for Your Neighbor," in which neighbors knock on each others' doors daily to check up on each other; "Sunshine" programs of regular visitations and "Hotline for the Aged," a telephone calling arrangement for consistent contacts.

Services for the Institutionalized Aged

Because of the severely restricted capabilities of the residents and the confining nature of a nursing facility, special recreational and adjunctive services must be provided for the institutionalized person. Rehabilitative and maintenance programs such as physical and occupational therapies and music, dance/movement, and art activities are becoming integral parts of the care of the confined elderly. The focus for the aged is on doing and being a contributing participant rather than a passive recipient.

Future Training Needs

The newly established disciplines of gerontology and geriatrics are growing rapidly to keep pace with the enormous increase in the proportion of elderly in our population. A survey has shown that 1275 schools offer at least one course in gerontology and the outlook is for continued government aid for training programs. The demand for professionals in the field will accelerate over the next 10 years with estimates of 1000 additional psychiatrists, 2000 clinical psychologists, 4000 psychiatric social workers, and 10,000 other specialists, in addition to medically trained staff members, required to provide services for the aged (8).

Because of the intent of Titles III and VII of the Older Americans Act and Title XX of the Social Security Act, there has been a general upgrading of program offerings and improved staff training in all publicly supported and licensed geriatric facilities. The American Hospital Association noted at their conference in 1971, "Winds of Change," that " . . . medicare . . . is recommending that extended care facilities provide the appropriate diversional programs directed by a qualified staff member." This indicates a " . . . long-overdue recognition of the fact that activities should be part of the health care plan and that they have value just as nursing, physical therapy, dietary, and all other services do" (9).

BACKGROUND OF THERAPEUTIC MOVEMENT FOR GERIATRICS

Historical Development of Therapeutic Dance

The roots of dance therapy may be found in ancient times in the tribal rituals of almost every pretechnological society. Primitive peoples have always sought physical means to communicate with the supernatural and to heal their spiritual ills. Rhythmic and symbolic movement has provided expression for people's fears and joys throughout the centuries.

Dance therapy, as we know it today, is a relatively new field that began about 30 years ago at the end of World War II. At that time, because of the extensive use of drugs for mental and emotional illness, it was necessary to find non-verbal therapeutic methods to reach the mentally ill patients. Two pioneers who utilized the improvisational self-expression processes of modern dance as an adjunct to psychotherapy at that time, were Marion Chace of Washington, D.C., and Blanche Evan of New York City. Their work, in very different settings and from uniquely personal viewpoints, provided therapeutic experiences involving group interaction, individual expression, and heightened body awareness for the participants.

From that beginning, dance therapy has developed into a tool for defining and directing individual progress toward well-being (sense of comfort, adjustment, and fulfillment) and has become an independent form of nonverbal therapy.

The American Dance Therapy Association was established in 1964 with Marion Chace as its first president. Since that time the profession has worked to establish standards for training and practice that include certification or "registry" for clinical therapists and has encouraged scholarship and research through journals and regular national and international conferences. The development of academic programs for undergraduate and graduate level college degrees in dance therapy is a fairly recent indication that the field is being recognized and accepted by colleagues in the "helping" professions.

At this time, action at the governmental level is taking place to promote the necessary funding and administrative organization for jobs and programming in dance therapy. Individual leaders in the field are making their work and their needs known to the public. The other creative arts therapies, art, music, and drama, together with dance, have joined forces to bring their message to Washington and the state capitals.

It is now acknowledged that dance therapy is effective in the treatment and conduct of programs for individuals with a wide range of physical and mental problems. Emotionally disturbed children and adults, institutionalized psychiatric patients, the physically handicapped, the elderly, and the learning disabled have all benefited from the use of dance/movement therapy. Therefore, in the 1970s dance therapy has achieved an equal status with the other health related professions.

Definition of Dance Therapy

Dance therapy is the use of rhythmic movement as a means of self-expression and communication that aids in the healthy integration of mind and body. The motivation to treat or improve the well-being of the participants is essential to the therapeutic character of the activity.

The concepts of modern dance, which utilizes movement improvisation with its relationship to time, space, and energy, laid the groundwork for the therapeutic use of dance. Dance therapy applies the interrelationships of movement elements, such as the amount of energy, type of flow, pace of action, and use of space to gain insight into the personality of the individual and to provide outlets for expression and socialization.

Special Needs of the Aging for Dance Therapy

Because the aging process is characterized by the onset of physical limitations and emotional stresses, it is vital to find outlets for self-expression and opportunities for social interaction, physical activity, and relaxation techniques. "The buildup of tension in the elderly can produce such symptoms as insomnia, fretfulness, and restlessness. The elderly often turn inward upon themselves their unrealised aggressive tendencies. These become a self-destructive force, leading to depression, which in turn, may increase tendencies toward psychosomatic diseases or lead to sudden outbursts of rage" (10). In addition, the normal process of disengagement, which takes place as one ages, is often accompanied by abnormal responses of withdrawal and depression that may be ameliorated through movement activity and the leader's guidance.

Dr. Paul Schilder, an English authority on body image and ego development, notes that "Movement is a great uniting factor between the different parts of one's own body" (11). He emphasizes the benefits of sensation and perception through which a person becomes aware of his/her relationship to the outside surroundings. Opportunities for movement provide experiences through which an individual can build a more accurate body image.

Geriatric movement sessions help participants to discover pleasure in moving and through that, to find pleasure in living. According to J. B. Helm and K. L. Gill, " . . . such programs (dance therapy), if effectively supported, can have a significant effect in reducing the resident population of our mental institutions, as well as improving the quality of life for our elderly" (12).

Purposes of Therapeutic Movement Sessions for the Elderly

Therapeutic movement sessions are ideally offered to discover, prevent, arrest, and reverse the damaging effects of aging. Opportunities to express emotions, both positive and negative, and to release tensions through movement experiences are invaluable parts of the therapeutic session. The movement therapist also offers stimulation for constructive recall, reality contacts, and social interaction. We are working to promote a freer relationship between body and mind by encouraging affirmative and meaningful gestures and movement.

The physical activity of the program produces the development of improved body alignment, increased range of motion, and relaxation for the reduction of stress. If we increase the range of movement and give opportunities for more physical experience, we are helping to increase the capabilities and therefore the individual's feelings of self-worth. Regular body exercise, according to Drs. Hans and Sulomach Kreitler (13), can provide emotional satisfaction. It can break the vicious cycle in which body image distortions caused by inactivity lead to more inactivity and further distortions. It can expend energies that need to be released and prevent internalization of aggression. Herbert A. de Vries has stated that even low intensity exercise, such as rhythmic movement activities, may have physiological benefits for muscles and joints (14).

The potentials of dance therapy for the aging are so far-ranging in scope because dance is unique as a therapeutic tool. The aesthetic and creative elements make it possible to integrate the body, mind, and spirit and so improve the substance of one's life.

UNIQUE APPROACHES WITH GERIATRIC CLIENTS

Special Therapeutic Viewpoint Toward Geriatric Groups

Working with the elderly differs from working with other groups in that we do not necessarily think of long-term goals, but instead work for immediate responses and improvement of the ability to cope with present problems. Isolation, dependency, and loss of identity are the most crucial concerns for the dance therapist to address when working with the aged.

It may be difficult to care for people who have offensive breath, watering eyes, and deformed bodies. One must resist the easy way of ignoring or rejecting the misery that is sometimes manifested. Great understanding and dedication are necessary to look past the argumentative, slow-moving, irrational, or unresponsive behavior and reach out to the human qualities and needs.

The older person is particularly sensitive to a patronizing, authoritarian leader so therapeutic sessions concentrate on giving and sharing. The group members are encouraged to be relaxed and free in a session that is not bounded by rigid expectations. Individual responses are accepted nonjudgmentally and each participant has the right to refuse or reject an activity. An essential element in this caring situation is acceptance through physical touch.

The elderly respond well to a slower, sometimes less active approach with much repetition. Gentle, but firm encouragement is essential. The limited expectations for the aged do not negate the great potential successes. For the dance therapist and the geriatric client, the rewards are in the smiles, the sparkling eyes, the outward signs of radiant joy, and a renewed participation that may be inspired by the movement session.

Differences Between Physical Therapy, Exercise Sessions, and Therapeutic Dance/Movement

There are overlapping elements in all modalities that utilize physical movement and so the goals, emphasis, and/or personal biases may account for some differences in content or presentation.

Many programs of physical exercise for the aging emphasize physical fitness and thus concentrate on cardiorespiratory efficiency. Dance/movement therapy sessions include activity that is more relevant to the development of improved body alignment and relaxation. They provide opportunities for emotional release and social interaction. Exercise that raises the heart rate less than 40% (rhythm and dance primarily) is not offered for conditioning purposes and yet the physiological benefits may be significant (15).

Physical participation is usually the sole purpose of the physical therapy and exercise sessions, whereas dance therapy also provides the opportunity for emotional reactions and insights. Sensitive and reflective comments or questions from the leader, and statements, gestures, or queries from the participants, are ways in which the session is incorporated into one's personal awareness.

Physiotherapy is often a required and nonvoluntary part of a patient's care which, although undeniably beneficial, may be uncomfortable or even painful. Dance/movement activities are informal and for the most part involve personal choice and individual expression in the free, rhythmic participation of the session. The emphasis is on pleasure and enjoyment. A highly respected British music therapist, Ruth Bright, has noted that " . . . restorative exercises (which are resisted when presented as rehabilitation per se) are performed enthusiastically when presented as a game or an action song" (16).

The geriatric dance therapist does not work primarily to develop specific skills but to encourage broader concepts and insights. For example, the physical therapist and the dance therapist both utilize the action of the arm forward and upward, but the physical therapist emphasizes the increased range of motion achieved and the dance therapist strives to develop the self-pride and the personal significance that comes with that accomplishment.

Criteria for Selection of Content

Various movement disciplines such as modern dance, folk dance, and ballet are used, but the emphasis is not on the technique or performance, but on the totality of the session itself. Many of the dance patterns are modified so that they are no longer in their original form, but the essence that is retained is valid, effective, and relevant for the participants.

In geriatric dance sessions the content may include instruction and recreational activities but the goals are not learning and enjoyment, even though both occur. Instead the emphasis is on the enrichment of each person's life for the optimum personal fulfillment.

Selecting activities and rhythmic accompaniment is influenced by knowledge of the clients' ethnicity, physical abilities, past experiences, religious preferences, and other such essential aspects of personal identity. An example of the advantages gained from appropriate offerings is this anecdote of one of our nursing home clients.

> I noticed Mrs. S. immediately at our first session. She was the only person who was not neatly dressed. Her hair was uncombed, her dress was torn, and her stockings were hanging loosely. She looked disoriented. The rest of the group treated her with disdain and a few told her to go back to her room. She was obviously the outcast. However, as soon as the music started, she stood up and started dancing by herself, completely unaware of her surroundings. When I held her hand she danced with me and wanted to do so continuously. Later, we danced in a circle and she stayed close to me and held my hand. The others did not want her in their circle. She never uttered a word, nor was there any vocal or facial response. She seemed lost in her own world. This participation was repeated at three more sessions. At the fifth one I put on a Yiddish record, "Lomer Alle Zingen" (a humorous song) and when she heard the word "kaptzonim" (which means poor people) she started laughing and repeating the word. Then she recited some of the other words in the song. As the music continued, she spoke to me and called me "darling." After that session she was friendly and warm toward me. The social worker told me she would not leave her room except for dance sessions. She is now a regular participant in our dance therapy group, but still spends the majority of her time alone in her room. Her verbal contacts (which started with the Yiddish recording) in our program seem to be her only social activity.

Necessity for Clarification of Goals

The therapist sets certain sociopsychophysical goals and tries to achieve them through the dance/movement program. It is necessary for the therapist-leader to have an agreement on goals with the administration of the facility and/or with the client and also to have a contract with oneself to facilitate a change in the group members. The ideal situation is to make a contract among all three parties concerned. This may be very simple and even informally agreed to, but sincerely accepted. If the program participants and the sponsors are able to identify realistic goals and agree to tackle them, then there will be more motivated cooperation. Then the sessions will not be "time fillers," but will produce the change essential to successful therapy.

Goals of the Older Adult for Rhythmic Activity Programs

Elderly persons are motivated to participate in dance/movement programs by physical and social benefits. They look forward to improved circulation in their legs, decrease of painful tensions, and the alleviation of labored breathing. The desire for physical comfort and greater flexibility is often the initial motivation for geriatric group members. After one or two sessions, the incentives to socialize and the opportunities to ease the monotony and loneliness of their daily lives become equally important. Almost every therapeutic movement session that we have led is highlighted by a participant saying such things as, "I feel so much better now than I did when I came in"; "You made me forget my pain"; "It's so good to be moving and feeling together!"; "I'm glad I didn't stay home alone again today"; and "I feel like you oiled the hinges of my body."

Therapeutic Goals of the Professional for Geriatric Dance/Movement Programs

Specialists in the fields of gerontology and medicine have noted that regular movement sessions help to stabilize or improve many mental, physical, psychological, and social functions of the aged. Psychogeriatrics specialist Dr. Brice

Pitt cites the importance of social interaction including dancing, "percussion sessions," and "keep fit" activities for the fun and physical benefits that are derived (17).

The treatment goals of the various therapies (recreational, occupational, music, and art therapies) for hospitalized patients were enumerated by Charlotte Green Schwartz and Elizabeth Rosen (18) as follows:

1. Increase socialization (develop interpersonal relationships).
2. Facilitate sublimation (redirect expression of primal drives into socially acceptable channels).
3. Alter self-attitudes (restore self-confidence and sense of security).
4. Develop new skills and interests (divert attention from personal symptoms).
5. Aid in adjustment to reality.
6. Assist staff understanding of patients' problems.

Specific functions and characteristics of the elderly that have shown improvement due to therapeutic dance activity and may be incorporated in the goals of the leader-therapist are listed below:

MENTAL	Memory	
	Alertness	
	Reality orientation	
	Judgment	
PHYSICAL	Circulation	Muscle tone
	Elimination	Coordination
	Sleep habits	Joint flexibility
	Respiration	Cardiac function
	Weight normalization	Body alignment and stance
	Digestion	Muscle strength

PSYCHOLOGICAL	Personal insight	Anxiety release
	Emotional stability	Realistic body image
	Latent feelings	Self-esteem
SOCIAL	Adaptability	Responsiveness
	Cooperativeness	Acceptance
	Verbal and nonverbal communication	
	Interpersonal relationships	

The positive effects of therapeutic dance/movement sessions are carried over to other activities and adaptive behaviors. We have received reports of the more active participation in arts and music programs and the improved response to meals and social events of our group members. They have become more cooperative in their lives when they have opportunities to participate in therapeutic movement activities.

CHARACTERISTICS OF THE GERIATRIC POPULATION

Chronological age is not an indication of the condition or outlook of an individual. We know of people in their fifties who are "old" because they have lost interest or reason for living. And we are acquainted with others in their eighties whose enthusiasm and appreciation of the world around them keeps them from being a geriatric stereotype. There is a natural, inescapable process of aging that begins at the moment of maturity and can be slowed down, accepted with grace, or confronted with rage. It is the adaptive techniques of the individual that makes it possible to cope with the problems of advancing years. Dr. Walter G. Klopfer has formulated a theory of the significance of interpersonal relationships to the aging process. He studied the adaptive techniques of disengagement, participation, and self-denigration that are most frequently used by the aged. Evidence seems to bear out the frequency of more positive adjustments to the aging process when people have opportunities for positive social experiences (19).

The Aging Syndrome

The physical and psychological regenerative processes slow down with individual variations to produce the following signs of the aging syndrome:

> Progressive loss of organ system function contributes to decreased motility and energy.
>
> Chronic organic disease often results in partially or totally disabling mental impairment.
>
> Societal expectations and pressure cause the greatest impairment of physical and mental function with regard to a positive outlook for the individual.

Physical Manifestations of Aging

One of the characteristics of the aging population is the physical manifestation of isolation and withdrawal. The range of movement is narrowed and the self-image is diminished. Actions become constricted and the viewpoint is introverted. Lack of attentiveness may result from turning off the outside world and focusing on personal needs and memories.

Another common sign of advanced age is a distorted body image that results in poor balance, ungainly gestures, and lack of confidence in physical abilities.

Additionally, the stooped spine, shuffling gait, drooping shoulders, and sunken chest are the visible results of the lower energy levels of the older adult.

An observation of the posture and movement patterns

of some aged persons is that of dance therapist, Jeri Salkin: "The older a person is or the longer he has had a fixed posture and way of moving, the more he becomes simple, obvious, immovable, abstract, and more like a caricature" (20).

Physical Limitations

Many disabilities of the aged are due not only to disease, but also to poor postural and mechanical use of the body. The spine is the symbolic lifeline of the body. The resiliency and alignment of the spine are true indicators of age in terms of mobility. The person whose regular movement patterns involve slumping, undue strain, and imbalanced use of the back will, with advancing age, develop severe restrictions and limitations of movement range. A good example of this is the actor who portrays an aging person by use of a rounded spine, small steps, and an irregular staccato pace for his walk. Many elderly persons are also painfully aware of their decreased stamina or the fact that they have "shrunk" with age. Some will even feel as inflexible as their chairs. Therefore, it is very helpful to explain the relationship of the muscles and the spine to freedom of motion and well-being.

As a person ages, the ligaments lose their elasticity and the individual's energy levels also decrease. One no longer resists the pull of gravity as efficiently or provides for the free use of the muscles. Increased tension is needed to maintain balance with poor alignment of the head, trunk, and legs and so one tires more quickly using unnecessary amounts of energy.

Psychological Manifestations of Aging

Enforced or voluntary inactivity results in accumulated tensions that are stored in the muscles and may cause restlessness, irritability, and even insomnia.

The loss of independence, whether financial or social, may produce a loss of self-confidence that may result in self-pity, passivity, frustration, or resentment.

The elderly often turn their unrealized aggressive tendencies inward, producing depression that may lead to psychosomatic illnesses or outbursts of sudden anger. Alternately, the aged person may resort to delusion or regression in an effort to withdraw from a too-painful reality.

Cerebral arteriosclerosis and other vascular and neurological diseases cause the destruction of brain cells resulting in chronic brain disease found in the geriatric population. This mental disorder causes such personality changes as anxiety, withdrawal, confusion, depression, hyperactivity, irrational actions, incontinence, forgetfulness, anger, and complaining or demanding behavior.

Characteristics of the Institutionalized Aged

The depersonalized atmosphere of many hospitals and nursing homes for the aged intensifies the disorientation in relation to time, person, or place, the extreme mood swings, loss of identity, and severe withdrawal of advancing age. Therefore it is essential to provide continual reinforcement, sensory stimulation, and to raise the energy levels of participants in geriatric sessions.

Specific Geriatric Physical Conditions

It is important to be aware of the variety and nature of physical limitations found in the geriatric population so that appropriate activities can be presented. The following are some of the common conditions caused by the progressive deterioration of the body during the aging process.

Circulatory disease: cardiac malfunction, hypertension, vascular disorders

Fractures: osteoporosis, accidents

Neurological impairments: stroke, arteriosclerosis, tumors, chronic brain syndrome

Impaired hearing

Reduced vision: cataracts, detached retina, diabetes

Amputation

Joint inflammation and restricted mobility: arthritis, bursitis

Muscle flaccidity: Parkinson's Disease, hypokineticism

Inadequate digestion and elimination: tooth loss, gum disease

We have discovered [as stated by Hirschberg, Lewis, and Thomas (21)], that many conditions caused by inactivity, such as pressure sores, muscle atrophy, certain circulatory problems such as hypostatic pneumonia, and even psychological deterioration, have responded to simple exercise done in bed or in a chair to a strong rhythmical accompaniment.

Chapter 2

ORGANIZATION OF THE GERIATRIC DANCE/ MOVEMENT PROGRAM

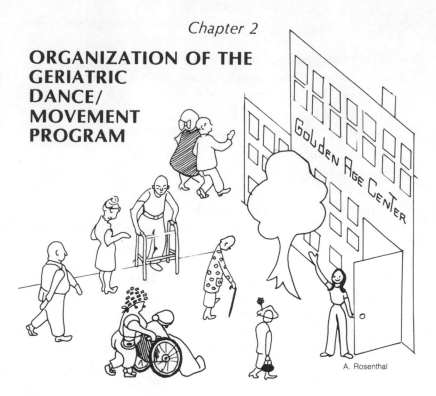

A. Rosenthal

GENERAL CONSIDERATIONS FOR ESTABLISHING A PROGRAM

Administrative Support

Due to recent legislation requiring the upgrading of program offerings and improvement of staff training in all public supported and licensed geriatric facilities, a new and increasing demand for enriched programming in recreational and therapeutic activities has emerged. Also, it has been noted by medical and administrative experts that when the elderly are physically active and socially involved, there is less need for medication and there are indications of sustained and improved daily functioning. Leaders have also cited that morale is improved for everyone, clients and staff, when therapeutic activities are successful. The dance/ movement program enlivens the whole atmosphere of the facility. Medical personnel, aides, and custodial employees can be seen responding to the music and activity by their smiles and bodily actions. Patients that are enjoyably occupied are easier to care for and become more cooperative. When staff observes the elderly responding to creative physical challenges, they are often impressed by their potential and with the universality of rhythmic response. Therefore, administrators of centers and institutions may well be receptive to the development of a therapeutic dance/movement program.

Ideally, the administrator will secure the services of a qualified geriatrics dance therapist, preferably one who is experienced and professional. If assistants or trainees are desirable, the program director should encourage them to participate on a regular basis with the approval of the leader-therapist.

It would be most helpful to enlist the active participation and cooperation of staff such as social workers, nurses, and other therapists. If possible, making the "rounds" or staff conferences available to the movement specialist would be highly beneficial to the patients/clients and the program. It would provide an opportunity for sharing and advising on new developments. Such involvement would also present the dance therapist to the clients as an adjunct to the treatment team.

Additionally, the administrator could schedule in-service workshops for staff members with the movement leader. The opportunity to participate in therapeutic movement sessions would offer insights into the goals of the program.

The program would also benefit from administrative assistance in circulating information about the dance/movement sessions and the sharing of positive results with doctors, nurses, social workers, volunteers, relatives, and visitors. This can be done through bulletin boards, newsletters, and other publicity outlets.

Responsibilities of the Geriatric Dance Leader-Therapist

In order to provide an activity program that is both therapeutic and recreational in scope, the responsibilities of the
leader-therapist should be to:

> Lead sessions.
> Give staff orientation.
> Keep records.
> Consult with the treatment team.

Diversity of Settings and Participants

Most settings for the elderly population include participants with different physical limitations and various ranges
of capabilities. Not only are the individuals diverse in their
personalities and physical abilities, but the situations in
which aged groups exist are extremely varied. They range
from recreationally oriented day centers for ambulatory,
independent older adults to therapeutic institutions cater-
ing to the infirm elderly. In each of these situations dance/
movement programs offer beneficial experiences.

We find large groups of older adults welcomed by local
community groups such as religious, civic, and social organizations that sponsor daytime drop-in centers with educational, recreational, and welfare programs. There is a great
increase in the number of retirement communities and residences for the elderly that provide leisure time activities
and cooperative personal development sessions. Movement programs that emphasize the recreational, social, and
physical well-being aspects are appropriate to these settings.

The activities personnel in rapidly proliferating nursing homes and hospitals are now responsible for a great
diversity of recreational-therapeutic planning in conjunc-

nming for
the institutionalized resident. In these situations dance/
movement sessions may be used as an adjunct to the physical and psychological therapies offered to maintain or improve the patient's status.

Medical Considerations

We suggest that a medical checkup or medical supervision
be provided, since all physical activity should be appropriate to the individual's physical condition, age, and psychological status.

Title for Dance/Movement Activity Sessions

Selecting a title that is appropriate for the group and the
setting is essential. Calling the sessions "therapy" or "therapeutic" may not be inviting to most older people, just as
encouraging someone to participate "because it's good for
you" is not always the best inducement. We have found that
emphasizing the enjoyment, relaxation, and well-being aspects of the program are more successful and accurate
descriptions. Some of the titles used for dance/movement
sessions in recreational and clinical settings are Exercise ·
with Music, Stay Healthy, Movement with Music, Dance-
Exercise for the Elderly, Rhythmics for the Retired, Experi-
encing Movement, Keep in Step, Exercise for Seniors,
Moving Together, Rhythmic Exercise, Fit and Fun Sessions, and Keeping Time. Any name that implies pleasure
and activity and is acceptable to the group would be an
asset to the program.

Size of Therapeutic Group

Dance/movement therapy with one client at a time is a
viable approach for many practitioners, but for the aged,

whether instit... ...nalized or comparatively independent
we advocate th... group setting. Certainly it is more econom-
ical to provide ... a group situation, and if the members are not
too heteroger... ...ous, there are other more important values
inherent in g... ...up activity. Interaction with... ...her ... ...ous
ages develop... ...ased empathy, a sense of inter...ersonal relationships, pe... support, and stimulation.

The nu...ber of persons in each ...erapy session may
vary from 3 to 30 and still be productive. The essential
criteria for s...ze of the therapeutic group are that the leader
can commu...cate with every person and that each group
member ca... be involved in the session. We have had the
most satisfy...ng groups with 10 to 16 people who are moderately limi...ed and with 3 to 6 severely disabled persons.
There are s...cessful programs for older adults that function with as many as 50 participants, but the therapeutic
goals are usually sacrificed for the recreational ones.

Scheduling of Sessions

Sessions are ideally scheduled on a regular basis in the
same space with the same personnel. A sense of stability
and continuity is essential to the development of trust and
comfort. If possible, individual sessions are most successful
when they are 45 to 50 minutes long. Regular, short periods of exercise are preferable to long, sporadic sessions.

Dance/movement sessions should be scheduled before rather than immediately after a meal, early in the day
before the onset of fatigue, and, if possible, at a time when
sedation or other medication is not needed at maximum
dosage.

Participation in the sessions will be greater if they are
not in competition with equally desirable activities. Participants should be prepared and assisted to attend the sessions in an unpressured atmosphere. We have discovered
that older adults join in more readily when they are invited

in their rooms or wards or in the dayrooms on their floors.

Program Reinforcement and Motivation

Another successful way to stimulate interest and enthusiasm in the ongoing program of movement activity, we
have found, is to prepare an album of anecdotes or photo-
graphs. Making a film or videotape or having sketches
drawn of participants, with their approval, provides a good
record. This kind of project establishes a tangible link
among group members and a concrete reality to be shared
with nonparticipants as a source of special pride in accomplishment.

Another way of sharing and offering recognition or
providing reinforcement for the group members may be in
the form of parties or open sharing sessions at the end of
a series. Participation in a program when outsiders or visitors may be invited to join in a favorite activity is often a
source of pleasure and fulfillment. We also recommend
small token gifts, badges, or attendance certificates to sig-

nify participation or appreciation for progress attained. Recognition and affirmation are gratefully accepted by everyone, but especially by the often neglected or patronized older person.

Record Keeping and Departmental Reports

It is most helpful to keep records of the content and progress of sessions and participants. Both the activities specialist and the program can benefit from well-kept records of the dance/movement sessions. Often recognition, acceptance, and support from institutional colleagues is a direct result of the opportunity to share specifics about one's work.

These notations can help the leader to plan future programs, chart and evaluate change in an individual's behavioral responses, and possibly even stimulate interest in further study or research.

Reports may be anecdotal in nature with brief references to significant changes in terms of an indicated time span. Or they may be outlines of participation in specific activities or the record of unusually successful or unsuccessful sessions. Examples of various kinds of record keeping are included elsewhere in this book.

QUALIFICATIONS FOR A GERIATRIC DANCE LEADER-THERAPIST

Training or Preparation

The most desirable preparation a geriatric dance therapist can have is diversified dance experience. A wide range of training develops personal ease and competence with movement, an extensive dance vocabulary, good rhythmic understanding, creative facility, and an uninhibited comfort about performing. The more styles and techniques of dance in which a prospective dance/movement leader has worked, the more flexible and responsive he/she can be to the therapeutic group.

Also, it is invaluable to include in one's training practice in observation skills, knowledge of movement behavior, group dynamics, and even neurophysiology. Certainly an understanding of the special problems of aging will be helpful in relating to and anticipating the group's needs.

Training, experience, and study will help leaders be alert to the special characteristics of the geriatric population and help them achieve the goals of the group rather than the ambitions or plans of the therapist.

The therapeutic dance/movement program may be led by specialists with varied primary training or certification. The geriatric dance leader-therapist may be a graduate of a master's degree program in dance therapy such as the one directed by Claire Schmais at Hunter College of the City University of New York in New York City. Or the leader may hold a degree in therapeutic recreation which includes courses in dance similar to the one taught by Linda Rocke at Suffolk Community College of the State University of New York on Long Island. Many competent movement leader-therapists are registered occupational or physical therapists or are persons who have completed study in gerontology or psychotherapy programs that included the application of expressive activities to the therapeutic process. Often the geriatric dance therapist has a rich background in dance performance and teaching and has also studied intensively through professional workshops and internships with dance therapists such as Eva Desca Garnet of Los Angeles, California and Susan Sandel of North Madison, Connecticut. Or the movement specialist has amassed extensive field experience with geriatric populations and has received training in effort shape analysis and movement observation techniques with experts such as Irmgard Bartenieff of the Laban Institute of Movement Studies in New York City. This diversified preparation often results in highly motivated and qualified personnel. Instead of standardized training which might produce narrowness of viewpoint or sterility of approach, the variety of backgrounds contributes to the continued enrichment and development of the field.

Personality Characteristics

Very special traits distinguish a successful leader of elderly groups. Primarily one is aware of the respect for the maturity and experience of the older adult through the manner in which meaningful activities and explanations are offered. The ability to establish an easy relationship with individuals and groups of the elderly may be based on a good combination of appreciation and empathy. A leader who is able to identify with the aging person and draw on pleasant, loving relationships and role models such as relatives, friends, and successful octagenarians will be able to establish a warm situation for growth and stability.

An important consideration when selecting a potential leader-therapist is to determine whether he/she is comfortable with physically or mentally disabled persons.

Personal attributes that make it possible to establish a relaxed, comfortable atmosphere are more conducive to productive movement sessions than the skills needed to present a well-organized lesson. Leading elderly groups require the ability to improvise and respond to diverse needs and to adjust to new and sudden demands. Therefore, the individual with a flexible personality is well-suited for this role.

The successful geriatric dance therapist has an optimistic outlook, is positive thinking, and is able to perceive situations in proper perspective. He/she is encouraging, pleasant, cheerful, and reassuring with an ability to accept differences or setbacks with a smile or a joke. A light touch with people and situations and a capacity for joy and the sharing of joyful experiences are ideal requisites.

Older people have particular needs for reassurance and security, since so much of their lives has been disrupted, changed, and often contains little positive future expectancies. Therefore, the dependability of the geriatrics activity leader is essential. Regularity of attendance, promptness, and careful planning provide a sense of form and balance that contributes to the beneficial aspects of the activity.

Technique of Presentation

The methods of presenting geriatric dance/movement sessions are distinguished by their informality. One is impressed with the friendly, sharing qualities of the leader and the development of an atmosphere of trust among the participants.

An inexperienced leader will soon find that the elderly participants limit themselves by their own awareness of strain, physical inability, or cautiousness. There is need for reasonable caution with demonstration and explanation, but extreme care should be taken to let the clients set the pace rather than the leader manipulating or forcing the individuals beyond their capacities. It will be more constructive to accept the spontaneous response that is forthcoming and to avoid projecting goals or standards. We have found it acceptable to both clients and program administrators if we present movement suggestions by saying, "Let's try this." And we preface any attempt to assist a client by asking, "May I take your hand?" or "Would you like me to touch your shoulder?" and so on.

An authoritarian attitude is not appropriate with elderly adults. One can be more effective by being sensitive to their needs, learning from them, sharing ideas, and recognizing what group members have to offer. Therefore, a leader who is too self-involved or concerned with his/her own image may not be able to relate with elderly groups.

In order to instill a sense of accomplishment and develop self-esteem, it helps to encourage rather than criticize. The leader who patiently waits rather than coaxes, and soothes instead of corrects, will find that the group members will react with trust and eagerness.

Because of the diversity of geriatric settings and participants, the leader therapist needs to use different approaches appropriate to each group. Sometimes it is essential to be dynamic and assertive in order to raise the energy levels. At other times the group members may need gentle, supportive leadership. Calm and consistent patience is particularly important when dealing with depressive or disoriented behavior. There have been many times when we have been grateful for an intuitively tactful response or a spontaneous assist from our sense of humor. We all strive to be the versatile therapist who can adjust the pace and tenor of a session to meet the unique needs of the situation.

If the leader acknowledges the members of the group as individuals with unique identities through the use of their names, then he/she is also contributing to reality orientation and positive self-image. Many aspects of institutionalized routine and the restrictions of age and finances deprive people of their identity. And so, the use of people's names and the recognition of their individuality are important therapeutic factors. We find that an essential basis of our work with the elderly is the belief in the uniquely precious qualities of each individual. We concentrate on the positive personality elements of our group members and their handicaps and deformities become less significant.

The conduct of a movement session is relaxed, but it does require successful, informal communication. Some suggestions can be presented by demonstration and physical participation, but verbal explanations are also significant sources of interaction. An audible, clear voice and simple, direct, nontechnical language are assets to a satisfying program.

Consideration of the leader's dress or appearance is often an intentional factor in the therapeutic presentation. A colorful, eye-catching outfit or interesting accessories may be a symbol of personal regard for the participants and produce a psychic lift for the whole group. Comfortable pants outfits or a smock or uniform that allows free action is most appropriate (rather than balletic or athletic outfits) for the geriatric movement therapist.

Facilities and Physical Environment

The facilities and physical surroundings in which the dance/movement program is offered will be determined by the varied situations that exist for the older citizens. Dayrooms, auditoriums, lounges, gymnasiums, and even corridors or the client's room may be used. If options are available, then consideration should be given to a well-lit and adequately ventilated, large area with a smooth and level floor. There should be a minimum of sight, sound, and other distractions. It is essential that the temperature of the room be moderate, approximately 70 degrees Fahrenheit, so that physical ease is assured.

The elderly, because of the often restricted nature of their present social contacts and limited range of mobility, are particularly sensitive and appreciative of color, design, and variety in their surroundings. This is especially true of the activities room. It has been noted that cheerful colors and neat and simple furnishings make people feel calm and more willing to participate in activities requiring energy and space utilization.

The room should be located where it will not disturb quieter activities, but also will not be isolated. The leader must be aware of the location of toileting and housekeeping facilities and procedures to secure emergency nursing services.

Chairs that are sturdy, movable, and with firm backs should be provided. If possible, provisions should be made to store or position wheelchairs, walkers, canes, and crutches so that participants can have the freedom or support that is necessary. (Also try to check to be sure that wheelchairs are locked before beginning seated activities.) The space available should accommodate sitting and/or standing arrangements so that everyone can see and even touch each other, if desired. This will help provide a sense of warmth and community.

When there are clients who can participate in reclining activity or relaxation, then padded, lightweight mats for floor work are necessary. (Carpet runners or foam pads may be used.)

An important adjunct to the dance/movement program is musical accompaniment. A record player that is simple and speed variable, plus a table for recordings, musical instruments, and other equipment are recommended furnishings for the dance activities room. In addition, the leader-therapist may appreciate a convenient, secure storage place between sessions.

Role of Aides or Assistants

Ideally, an assistant should be available to help with the phonograph, distractions such as telephones or visitors, and with the personal needs of group members. Activities personnel, aides, or volunteers can be great assets to the program if they are responsive to the direction of the leader. It is helpful if they participate unobtrusively and are willing to distribute and collect instruments and props. They may be appreciated as partners or as additional leaders when asked by the leader-therapist.

Nurses and aides who assist with groups may need to be advised that immediate participation or overt response should not be anticipated or overreacted to. Sometimes there are tendencies to remove a person who doesn't seem alert or responsive. Patients may really be benefiting from passive observation or may need time to feel comfortable in a situation. Also we have not found it helpful when too much attention or enthusiasm is directed by assistants toward individual participants. This is especially undesirable when self-involvement or group-directed activity is the objective.

We have benefited from the assistance of nursing aides, therapy student-interns, and volunteers who pushed wheelchairs, held boxes, changed recordings, and moved with great sensitivity along with the group members.

Staff members who join in the sessions may be able to provide some reinforcement or carryover to other activities in between group meetings. These assistants may also contribute another viewpoint to the record keeping and evaluation of the therapeutic dance/movement program.

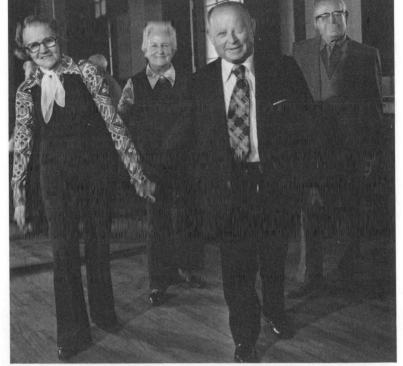

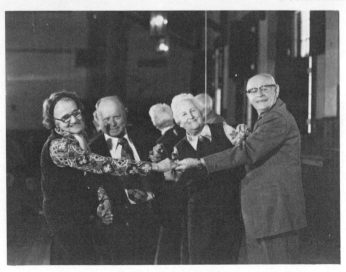

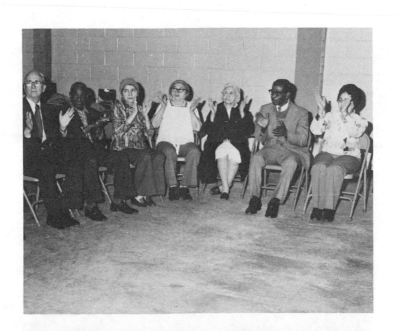

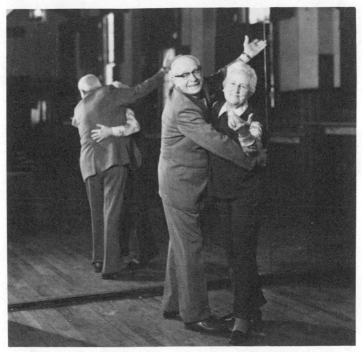

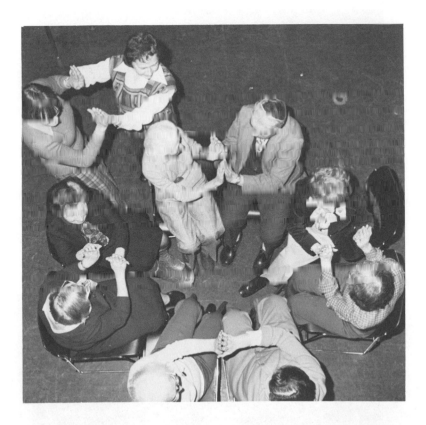

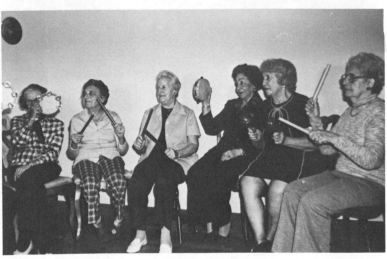

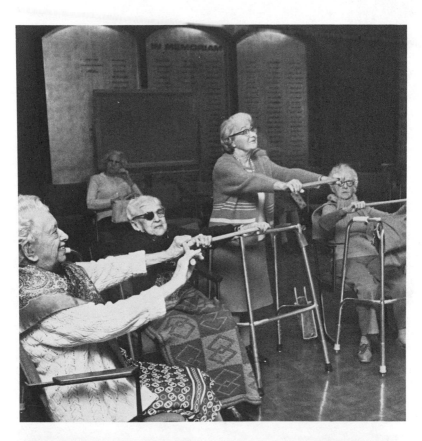

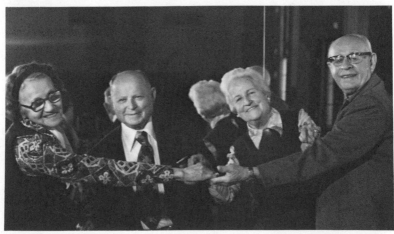

Chapter 3

GENERAL OVERVIEW OF THE SESSION

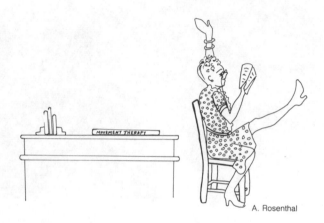

A. Rosenthal

VALUE OF STRUCTURE FOR THE SESSION

A planned structure is essential to the geriatric movement session because it provides security, stability, and assurance for the participants. It also reinforces a sense of self-worth and accomplishment by providing a form for individual and group efforts.

Structure is like choreography in the manner in which one builds and releases energy and uses rhythmic, physical activity with the emotional component. This physical program utilizes creative imagery and personal expression through patterned body movement.

BASIC FORMAT

The ideal geriatric dance/movement session is comprised of four parts: the opening, the warm-up activities including sequential exercises (interspersed with some massage and breathing), the creative or expressive dance patterns, and the quiet period of relaxation and summation. The session with its variety of pace, style, and range of movement offers stimulation, relaxation, and emotional release as needed.

There are many ways of shaping or forming a therapeutic session, from the most nondirective experiential ones to those involving highly structured components. Each may have value when serving the specific needs of the participants. Variations of format may also depend on the size of the group and the limits of time and space. According to the specifics of the group or the agency in which the program is established, one or another aspect of the session may be emphasized; or the order in which they are presented may be changed. With some groups the creative, nondirective activities are more important and comprise the entire session. This is particularly true with groups where there is a wide diversity of physical ability. Alternately, when working with elderly adults who are ambulatory and physically able, the leader can initiate more energetic and challenging physical movement patterns. With most groups, a low-status type of leadership is essential for individuals to express themselves freely.

A circle formation is especially effective to provide a feeling of acceptance and equality of opportunity. It also establishes a form that allows for contact or distance between members and a space to move in or out of. The circle is a symbol of protection and unity that helps create an atmosphere of trust and comfort for the group.

There are basically two different leadership techniques used in working with geriatric movement groups. One emphasizes the analysis of movement and its relationship to

the individual's needs. This usually involves careful explanations and verbal accompaniment for the movement activity. The other approach involves participation in a
mirrorlike experience between leader and group. This utilizes rhythmic accompaniment with minimal vocal cues
from the leader, who might be the professional therapist or
a member of the group. The two approaches may be used
independently or in combination. For example, withdrawn,
extremely depressed groups of senile will benefit most
from the stimulation of music. A more alert and active
group will appreciate developing an understanding of their
activities. Therefore, a rule might be that the less alert the
geriatric group is, the less explanation is appropriate.

The leader-therapist plans a general outline for each
session. Every well-balanced session will include activities
that are specifically selected to enhance the total person,
including the physiological, psychological, emotional, and
social development. These activities are most successful
when they are relevant to the participant's life experiences
—past, present, and future. This is the basic format, but the
response and interaction of each individual and the combined "chemistry" of the group create their own quality
and substance.

SPECIFIC SUGGESTIONS FOR SESSION ORGANIZATION

The format of each session is planned to include at least
one activity in which the leader-therapist participates in a
one-to-one relationship, that is, offers special individual
attention with some of the group members. Throughout
the activity period both unison and small groups or individual participation is encouraged.

When working with older adults, it is advisable to
present a few movement suggestions rather than "jam

packing" the session and thus overwhelming or producing superficial results.

Memory spans may be short and so there should be repetition without expectations of conscious carryover from session to session. It is also helpful to repeat material so that an adequate level of proficiency is achieved. This will give the individual confidence in his/her ability. When the leader builds upon simple achievements the group remains enthusiastic and is willing to venture into new experiences.

Advance planning for each session should include more ideas and activities than might be used so that there are options to choose if necessary. With elderly groups the dance therapist quickly becomes aware of whether the material presented is suitable or not. Geriatric clients do not usually feel obliged to conform to social expectations. If they don't find the activity satisfying, they will leave or withdraw.

Often a particular question or response may offer a new direction for the session. Also presentation of subjects relating to the personal needs of the aged or discussions of problems about movement will sometimes reveal areas of concern that can be dealt with in the session or may be referred to the other members of the treatment team. The leader, therefore, must be sensitive and flexible for this potential. Recognition of these special sparks often provides the magic glow for moments that produce real change and growth even in the aged individual.

SUGGESTED APPROACHES FOR SPECIFIC DISABILITIES

Amputation—encourage use of remaining limbs; adapt movement sequences for either legs or arms or one part alone

Arthritis—concentrate on increasing circulation and flexibility in joints through relaxation, massage, and gentle, smooth movement progressions

Blindness—offer more touch and physical contact, present less space-oriented activity with more verbal instructions; use clearly accented music accompaniment

Deafness—clarity simplicity, and slow-paced verbal instructions accompanied by demonstration is essential; avoid shrill, high-pitched and particularly loud, pounding sounds

Hypertension—emphasize the relaxing elements of movement

Neurological impairments—offer individual help or special couple activities in which people work together or with leader; use unaffected limb to assist weaker or paralyzed part

Senility—patiently encourage participation in simple activities; work for attention and sense of accomplishment; pleasurable involvement can arrest or reverse progress of senility

GUIDELINES FOR THE LEADER-THERAPIST

In order to create an atmosphere that is relaxed, comfortable, and contributes to a joyful experience, the leader may find these suggestions for presentation helpful.

1. Lead or conduct the sessions, rather than teach the activities. The leader-therapist shares in the experience of the group.
2. Encourage participation, rather than imitation, by presenting movement sequences or ideas and accepting the responses of the participants.

3. Communicate on the level of the participants. Use imagery and vocabulary that is acceptable and in harmony with their expressed wishes. Respect the age and past accomplishments of individuals and treat them accordingly.

4. Remind the group of improvement and changes noted. Describe the goals of various activities; point out the positive effects of the session and the benefits derived.

5. Make it a point to physically reach out and touch each member of the group as you sense that they will be receptive. Such contact provides reassurance, affirmation, sensual pleasure, and stimulation.

6. Be sensitive to the moods and reactions of group members. Reflect the actions and ideas expressed. Pick up nonverbal cues because the emotional and mental state of the individual is often reflected in his/her physical actions.

7. Keep the goals of the group members in mind so that participants are not exploited and manipulated for the leader's personal satisfactions.

8. Encourage individual questions and responses. This can be done before, during, or after the session. Be open and flexible about the "agenda" —the flow of a session is independent and should be guided, but not rigidly controlled.

9. Use compliments and encouraging phrases in order to develop positive self-image and reinforce self-esteem. Negative comments or criticisms of performance are not helpful for these groups. It is much more effective to compliment a successful attempt or to draw attention to the correct way.

10. Emphasize simplicity. Use specific language so

that the group is not overwhelmed with too many
stimuli or complicated patterns.

11. Anticipate whether specific directions for right or
left sides are appropriate or not. Clients may not
be able to respond to such instructions because
of physical, mental, or even emotional limitations. Also it can be confusing if the leader stands
opposite to a patient or in a circle with a group
when giving directions of right and left. Try to
stand next to one person or at the end or the
middle of a line of people if it is desirable to
specify right or left.

12. Have realistic expectations for your clients. Over-
estimating the capacities of the group may dis-
courage response, but moderate optimism will
usually elicit greater effort.

13. It is important to present ideas or suggestions on
an adult level that will appeal to mature interests.
Avoid talking down to group members in an
effort to achieve clarity and simplicity.

14. Voluntary participation is essential. Only gentle
encouragement, subtle invitations, or suggestions should be offered, with the option to withdraw or refuse always available.

15. Patiently observe clients' reactions instead of
pushing for verbal response. Among group members there may be a wide range in the ability to
communicate. Nonverbal communication is the
integral element of therapeutic movement. As a
master dance therapist, Jeri Salkin, said, ". . . for
the old . . . who are functioning in their own
world, it may be far more meaningful to touch,
feel, and to move than to listen, hear, and do"
(22).

16. Pace activities within the time span. Include vigorous and relaxing portions according to the

length of the session and the energy levels of the group. Invite people to rest or vary the movement as personal needs arise.

17. Periodically encourage clients to look at and accept each others' movements in order to develop an awareness and recognition of other people.

18. Use a good balance of repetition and variety. Do not use exactly the same patterns all the time, but retain satisfying ones.

19. Attempt to introduce material relevant to the "outside" or larger world for remotivation. Recognize holidays, seasons, and special events. Share personal views and experiences when appropriate.

20. Make provisions for the variety of physical and psychosocial disorders that may be present. The limited range of movement possible may make it necessary to confine most activity to the sitting position.

21. Offer a developmental program so that participants derive a sense of realistic challenge and accomplishment that is within their range of capabilities.

22. Use a moderate approach with physical exertion and emotional stimulation. Elderly people may be timid, frightened, or severely limited and infirm. Start with untaxing and nonthreatening movement and build as group responds. Avoid turning, spinning actions, sudden head motions, strongly percussive or propulsive gestures, unless initiated by the participant.

23. Sustain attention by using smooth transitions from one action to another.

24. Anticipate and provide a positive "closure" for the session. It is advisable to offer group members a shared or individual opportunity to feel

calm and satisfied with the completion of the period. Recognition of breathing rhythms (encourage slow, steady rate) facial expressions (calm or joyful), or body set (uplifted relaxed), will help guide the final activity of the participants.

PHYSICAL ACTIVITIES FOR THE THERAPEUTIC DANCE/MOVEMENT SESSION

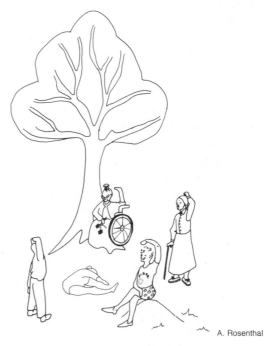

A. Rosenthal

THE OPENING (GREETING)

Sometimes the leader arrives before the participants gather and in other situations the group is already waiting when the therapist enters. Each of these beginnings may present different challenges for the opening or start of a productive session.

Ideally, the group should be arranged in a circle or semicircle formation. It has been found that some of the advantages of a circle are the development of group solidarity, wide range of visibility, and reduction of anxiety.

Playing strongly rhythmic, bright, and melodic music as participants enter is often a way of providing a psychic lift to enliven or "wake up" individuals. Because many of the patients may be sedated or heavily medicated, it may be necessary to offer an energetic, dynamic approach that will bring an immediate positive response. (See page 222 for suggested music for opening the session.)

It is essential to establish an initial contact with individuals to develop trust and rapport and to establish the desired mood of anticipation. A ritualistic or repetitious way of starting sessions provides continuity for the program. Shaking hands, arranging chairs, touching a shoulder or a cheek as the leader progresses about the room in an established order, standing at the door as each person enters, or "calling for" participants in a dayroom or ward may be the routine established.

The therapist should strive to set a tone of friendly, personal interest. Greeting the men and women and signifying concern over absentees or delight for returnees to the program will bring an immediate positive response.

Referring to past sessions is sometimes helpful, but should only be attempted with the understanding that aging often presents problems of time orientation and memory deterioration. References should be used with caution and a light touch.

Brief questions or discussion may take place during the opening part of the session, but an emphasis on physical participation should be encouraged as soon as possible.

MOVEMENT ACTIVITIES

Purpose of "Warm-up" Activities

The "warm-up" is usually the portion of the session right after the initial welcome or greeting. It is activity for general body involvement to raise the energy level, increase respiration, and stimulate circulation. According to Dr. Hans Kraus, an authority on therapeutic exercise, ". . . the aim of (general exercise) . . . is principally to produce changes; i.e. improvement of circulation, general muscle power, or general relaxation" (23). "With general exercises . . . the aim is to influence the whole organism: circulation, breathing, general muscle power, metabolism, and digestion" (24). Kraus believes that specific, local problems affecting certain muscle groups are relatively insignificant to the aim of improving the general condition of the patient.

Precautions Regarding Warm-up and Exercises

The medical limitations of group members must be known to the leader-therapist before beginning any physical activity session. Also, if possible, it would be helpful to be aware of the participants' previous experience with exercise and dance and to know any pertinent details concerning their weight, smoking habits, or medications.

Exercises should not be performed with stress and tension present. Increased flexibility and range of motion can be achieved with ease and comfort. An easy, slow, and thorough warm-up is especially necessary for geriatric groups.

Peripheral circulation (in hands and feet) should be encouraged, in addition to as much total body involvement as possible.

It is advisable to work within the guidelines of each agency regarding physical contact between staff and clients. Sometimes it is necessary to be wary of assistance that might be construed as manipulation. We have found that gentle cautiousness and waiting to follow the lead or request of the client are good ways to avoid exploitation and frustration.

Value of Diversity

The preparational warm-up should include body movement with variations of space, time, and energy. Space patterns of up and down, large and small, and side to side;
time variations of slow and fast and energy variations like
strong and weak are essential for a well-balanced program.

To increase the movement range and abilities of the
aged individual, encourage them to extend and flex their
bodies in as many directions and different levels as possible. The use of the natural rhythm of swinging in which the
weight of the body gives in to the pull of gravity develops
balance and provides the experience of the interaction between control and release.

The energy levels of the lethargic or depressed person
may be raised by stimulating circulation and respiratory
rate with slapping, clapping, and rubbing actions and by
changing the speed and force of the movements.

For warm-up and creative activities, incorporating the
eight basic actions as outlined by Rudolf Laban in his
Effort-Shape method and Audrey Wethered in *Movement
and Drama in Therapy* will provide the desired diversity (25):

1. Thrusting   (hammering and punching)
2. Pressing   (pushing and pulling)
3. Wringing   (unscrewing a tight jar lid)
4. Slashing   (cutting wheat or cracking a
                    whip)
5. Flicking   (brushing off dust)
6. Dabbing   (patting on powder)
7. Gliding   (smoothing a tablecloth or
                    ironing clothes)
8. Floating   (moving like a feather in a
                    breeze)

Warming up the body can be achieved by exercise
sequences or by movement exploration. Discovering the

area around one helps to tone up the total body and make one aware of the freedom and control of the individual's physical space. This helps to avoid mechanical directions of stretching and bending or flexing and extending.

Use of Imagery

Creative use of imagery and fantasy to encourage use of varied movement expression is helpful for the total involvement of the individual. Phrases such as "Try it as though . . .," "Let's imagine that . . .," "What if . . .?", and "Remember when . . .?" may be used. For example, many groups respond well when the leader says, "Stretch your arms up as if you're reaching for the sky or touching the stars" or "Remember when you used a sewing machine with a foot treadle? Let's lift our heels and toes alternately like that." Descriptive suggestions like a rocking chair or playground swing or a clock pendulum have been successful for initiating pleasant and even vigorous swinging actions. An imaginary tug-of war or pushing invisible pianos may inspire strong flexions and extensions of the arms and torso. Whenever such images are introduced, the group will have an opportunity of sharing the leader's experiences, the participation will take on richer dimensions, and group members may possibly offer creative stimuli of their own.

SUGGESTED SEQUENCES OF EXERCISE PROGRESSIONS

These sequences are not presented as rigid lesson plans. The leader-therapist should be sensitive and receptive to the moods and needs of the participants. This may necessitate such changes as elimination, additions, or variations in the suggested format. It is also important to pace the activity sequence so that the group does not strain or become overtired. No exercise should be repeated more than three times, unless the group is particularly energetic. Every three or four exercises may be interspersed with opportunities for slow breathing and relaxation. We also find that gentle self-massaging activities, (such as those of the face, hands, and knees), are good to introduce in between more energetic movements.

Four separate exercise series are offered for a diverse range of geriatric abilities. The activities can be varied by the leader in a more challenging or less demanding way as needed by changing the number of repetitions and the amount of energy used. Also movements from the various exercise sequences can be interchanged as judged appropriate by the leader.

Precise timing for the exercises is not stressed, since the pace will depend on the individual's strength, flexibility, and temperament. But we have found that rhythmic accompaniment and background music can give purpose and mood to the action. (See page 224 for suggested music for accompaniment.)

Energetic Activities For Active, Independent Older Citizens

These movement suggestions are for individuals who are within the parameters of normal physical health and range of mobility for their age.

(Exercises A through Q may be done standing or sitting.)

Exercise A.   Spinal Extension

Sitting forward in a chair, with feet firmly placed on the floor and the hands holding onto the sides of the chair, take four counts to take a deep breath, press down on the hands to straighten the spine. Then exhale with a hissing sound, letting the spine round and the abdomen draw in toward the spine for four counts. Repeat this two times. When you work with a group for consecutive sessions, then you can increase the exhalation to eight counts.

Exercise B.   Head and Neck Exercise (Figure 4–1)

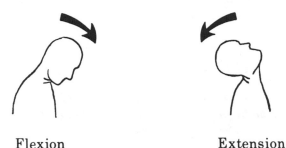

Flexion   Extension

Figure 4-1   Head and neck exercise. (From *Elementary Rehabilitation Nursing Care,* U. S. Public Health Service, Division of Nursing.)

Let the head fall forward to the chest and return to centered position four times. Let the head relax backward by lifting the chin and return to centered position four times. (You may add hands clasped at the back of head or neck.)

Exercise C.   Head Rotation (Figure 4–2)

Turn the head to the right so that the nose is over the right shoulder, then turn the head to the left shoulder. Repeat three times from side to side. (You may say "No" at the same time.)

Exercise D.   Head Circle

Gently and slowly let the head fall forward bringing the chin to the chest. Then turn chin toward right shoulder, let the head go backward, turn chin in toward left shoulder, and return head to centered position. Repeat once in opposite direction.

Turning head to look over the shoulder

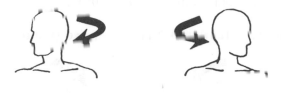

Right rotation   Left rotation

Figure 4-2   Head rotation. (From *Elementary Rehabilitation Nursing Care,* U. S. Public Health Service, Division of Nursing.)

Exercise E.   Swimming Action

Do the Australian swim crawl action with the arms alternately extending and flexing in front of body in large strokes six times.

Exercise F.   Punching

Alternately thrust one arm forward with fist clenched at shoulder level four times and thrust upward toward ceiling four times. Repeat four counts for each arm punching in each direction.

Exercise G.   Pushing and Pressing

Use arms to push imaginary windows open then use arms to press them closed.

Exercise H.   Eye Exercises Around the Clock

Move the eyes in a circle clockwise one time and counterclockwise one time as though following the numbers around a clock face.

Exercise I.   Rubbing Hands and Cupping Eyes

Rub the palms of the hands together briskly until they feel warm. Then place the palms of the hands cupped over the eyes and keep that position for a moment.

Exercise J.   Facial Exercise

Exaggeratedly mouth the vowel sounds A E I O U so that the face is activated.

Exercise K.   Elbow Circling

With elbows bent and hands at shoulders, circle the elbows forward, upward, backward, and downward. Make three or four circles with both arms.

Exercise L.   Chest Expansion and Arm-Shoulder Extension—Wings Open and Close

With elbows bent and hands at shoulders, bring the elbows backward and then return them to starting position. Then extend arms at shoulder height toward the back and then bend elbows and return to starting position. Alternate elbow and arm motions two times.

Exercise M.   Spine Stretch

Lift the arms overhead as you inhale and lift the chest. Then extend the spine forward, extending arms diagonally toward floor. Relax the arms downward toward the floor and exhale while you lower head toward the knees. Slowly return to starting position.

Exercise N.   Arm Circles

Both arms circle—vary the size and the height of the circles from small and low toward the floor to larger and higher and back down to small again. The circles may be in front or at the sides of the body.

Exercise O   Lateral Torso Stretch (Figure 4-3)

Bending sideways from the waist.

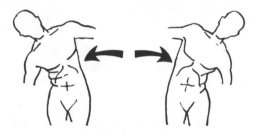

Figure 4-3   Lateral torso stretch. (From *Elementary Rehabilitation Nursing Care,* U. S. Public Health Service, Division of Nursing.)

Bend toward the right side, letting the right arm hang down at side as left arm is raised overhead. Return to starting position and repeat to the left side.

Exercise P.   "Zipper" Stretch

Raise the right arm overhead, bend the elbow, and touch the right hand to the back of neck. Bring left hand behind back with the elbow bent and try to clasp right hand with left hand. Repeat on opposite side.

Exercise Q. Half Spinal (Yoga) Twist (Figure 4–4)

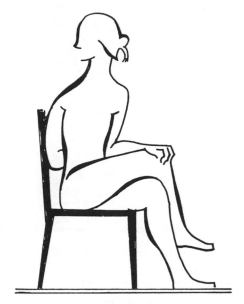

Figure 4-4   Half spinal (yoga) twist. Kassoy

Cross the right knee over the left and put the left hand on the right knee. Twist the torso to the right, turning the head to look over the right shoulder. Bring the right arm behind the body at the waistline. Repeat to the other side.

Exercise R. "Sit Up" (Figure 4–5)

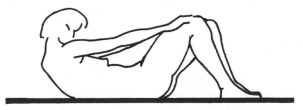

Figure 4-5   Modified sit-up. Kassoy

Lie on back with knees bent and feet placed close together on floor. Extend arms with hands resting on front of thighs.

Tighten abdominal muscles and bring head and shoulders forward close to chest, about six to ten inches off the floor while sliding hands along thighs toward the knees. Hold this curled position for approximately four counts and then slowly uncurl to starting position, placing shoulders and head on floor and relax.

Exercise S.   Side Leg Lifts (Figure 4-6)

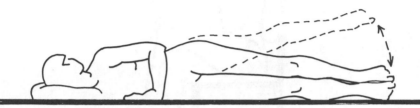

Figure 4-6   Side leg lifts. Kassoy

Lie on right side with right arm under head and left hand on floor in front of chest for support. Lift left leg up and return to starting position. Repeat four to eight times, depending on individual capacity. Repeat same on left side.

(Exercises T through X may be done seated or lying on back.)

Exercise T.   Knee-to-Chest Stretch

Clasp the hands around the right knee and raise the knee toward the chest three times with pulsing motion. Repeat with the other knee.

Exercise U.   Head-to-Knee Stretch

Lift right leg and bend the knee. Clasp the hands around the right knee and raise the knee toward the chest and lower the head toward the knee. Hold position for three counts. Then lower the foot to the floor and return the head to starting position. Repeat with breathing: Inhale when lifting the knee and exhale when head is lowered toward knee and lower leg to floor.

Exercise V.   Ankle Rotation (Circling)

Cross the right leg over the left thigh and circle the right ankle outward four times and circle the ankle inward four times. Repeat with the left leg crossed over the right.

Exercise W.   Leg Extensions

Starting with the feet together on the floor and with the knees bent, slide the feet together along the floor until the legs are extended. Then slide them apart to the sides and then close the extended legs together. Flex knees and return feet to starting position. Repeat three times.

Exercise X.   Scissors Kick

Extend both legs off the floor in front and alternately kick the legs up and down close together and quickly, like splashing.

(Exercises Y through AA may be done seated.)

Exercise Y.   Treadle Movement

Move the feet as if you were operating the treadle of an old-fashioned sewing machine. With one foot in front of the other, raise the toes and then the heels alternately.

Exercise Z.   Typewriter and Piano Movements

Using the fingers in individual lifting and lowering actions, imitate typing and piano playing movements on a huge imaginary keyboard.

Exercise AA.   Hand Movement

Lift the arms and wave hello and goodbye; shake the arms as though signaling the teacher.

(Exercises AA through GG may be done standing.)

Exercise BB.   Spine-and-Hamstring Stretch (Figure 4–7)

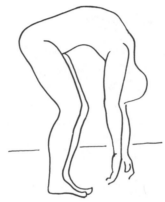

Figure 4-7   Spine-and-hamstring stretch. Kassoy

Let the head relax forward, bring chin to chest, allow head and neck to lead shoulders forward as spine relaxes. Bend forward from the waist and relax knees, if standing. Breathe slowly in and out while in forward relaxed position. Return to starting position slowly by uncurling from the lower back, then the upper torso, and finally the neck and head.

Exercise CC.   Wall Push (Figure 4–8)

Stand with feet parallel facing a wall with arms extended so that the hands may be placed at chest height on the wall. Bend elbows and lean body slowly toward the wall keeping the heels on the floor. Then push against the wall with the hands and press to return slowly to starting position.

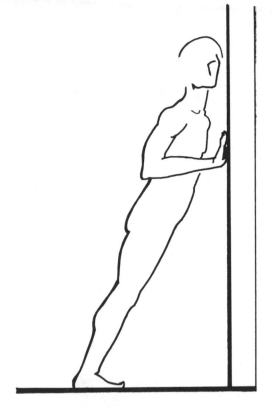

Figure 4-8   Wall push. Kassoy

Exercise DD.   Waist-and-Torso Rotation (Figure 4–9)

Place hands on waist and slowly twist torso alternately to the right and to the left sides four times.

Exercise EE.   Knee Bends (Figure 4–10)

Stand in back of a sturdy chair; hold onto the chair back with both hands. Bend the knees without taking the heels off the floor, then straighten knees to starting position. Repeat two times. Then do two more knee bends taking

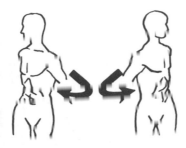

Right rotation   Left rotation

Figure 4-9   Waist-and-torso rotation. (From *Elementary Rehabilitation Nursing Care,* U. S. Public Health Service, Division of Nursing.)

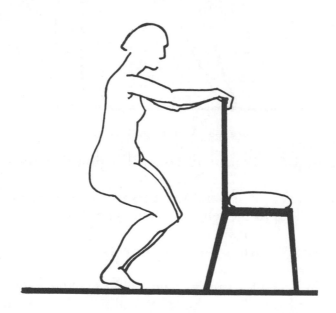

Figure 4-10   Knee bends. Kassoy

heels off floor in order to lower body a little more. Then in sequence, bend knees, straighten knees, lift heels and bring heels down. Repeat two times.

Exercise FF.   Relax by Shaking Legs

Alternately shake out legs, while hands hold onto chair for support.

Exercise GG.   Leg Swings (Figure 4–11)

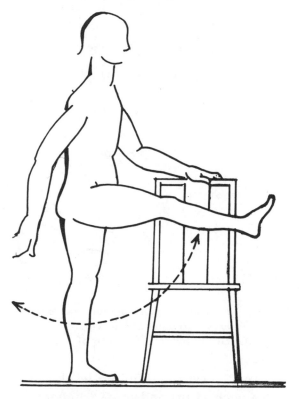

Figure 4-11   Leg swings. Kassoy

With left side of body facing the back of a chair, hold onto the chair with the left hand, swing the right leg forward and backward. Repeat on the other side.

Note: Energetic exercises should be done with discretion and should not necessarily all be used in the same session.

Moderate Activities For Partially Disabled and Relatively Restricted Older Persons

Exercise A.   Clapping and Circling Hands

Clap hands in time to music while raising arms to make a large circular path in front of body, first clockwise and then counterclockwise. About 16 counts can be used for each circle.

Exercise B.   Arm-and-Hand Flexion and Extension
(Figure 4–12)

Bending fingers toward palm (make a fist).
Returning fingers to neutral position (straighten fingers).

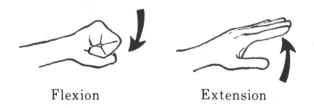

Flexion   Extension

**Figure 4-12   Arm-and-hand flexion and extension.
(From *Elementary Rehabilitation Nursing Care,* U. S.
Public Health Service, Division of Nursing.)**

Extend the arms forward at shoulder level, make fists and then stretch fingers. Curl and uncurl fingers four times, then make fists and draw elbows back close to chest as hands move toward shoulders in a pulling action. Repeat four times.

Exercise C.   Breast Stroke

Bend the elbows to the side with the hands in front of chest, extend the arms forward at shoulder level, and make a semicircle with the arms to the sides, then flex elbows and return the hands to starting position. Repeat four times.

Exercise D.   Shake Hands, Shoulders, and Arms

Shake hands in front of body. Relax arms at sides and shake the entire arm from the shoulders. With hands resting on knees, shake the shoulders.

Exercise E.   Eye Exercise

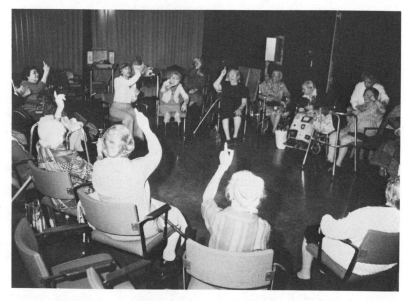

Photo 1   Eye Exercise
Benjamin B. Scherman

Extend one finger at arms length forward and watch it as you move it toward the tip of your nose. Then follow, with your eyes, as your finger moves to the right and then to the left. Do not move the head, only the eyes. Close eyes and rest. Repeat

Exercise F.   Hand Fan (Figure 4-13)

> Moving fingers apart (spread fingers)
> Moving fingers together.

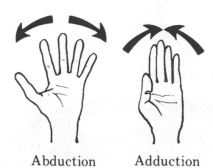

Abduction   Adduction

Figure 4-13   Hand fan. (From *Elementary Rehabilitation Nursing Care,* U. S. Public Health Service, Division of Nursing.)

Place the hands together (in praying position) and then slowly make spaces between fingers by spreading them apart and then close them, like a fan.

Exercise G.   Flying Movements (make sure there is sufficient space between participants)

With arms at sides of body and palms facing inward, lift both arms sideward to shoulder level with wrists relaxed and then lower arms. Exercise may be varied by using one arm at a time or alternately lifting and lowering the arms like wings.

Exercise H.   Shoulder Exercise

Move shoulders up and down and then backward with the arms hanging relaxed at the sides.

Exercise I.   "Yes"-And-"No" Head and Neck Movements

With large movements extend and flex neck muscles so that head moves horizontally and vertically, nodding "yes" and "no."

Exercise J.   Mouth Motions

Chew a large, imaginary piece of meat like a lion or tiger would, making exaggerated faces as the jaw opens and closes. Say "prunes" and "cheese" and feel the mouth and cheeks shape the words.

Exercise K.   Head-and-Neck Exercise

Drop the head forward toward chest and move head to the right shoulder, keeping chin down move head back to center, then move head to the left shoulder; keeping the chin down, move it back to center. Raise head to upright position.

Exercise L.   Head-and-Neck Exercise (Figure 4–14)

Begin with the head in an upright position and tilt head so that the right ear moves toward the right shoulder. Then relax head and neck to the left so that head tilts the left ear toward the left shoulder.

Bending head so that ear is moved toward shoulder.

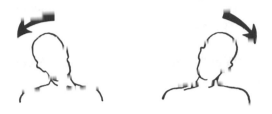

Right lateral flexion   Left lateral flexion

Figure 4-14   Head-and-neck exercise. (From
Elementary Rehabilitation Nursing Care, **U. S. Public
Health Service, Division of Nursing.)**

Exercise M.   Shoulder Shrugs

Place hands on shoulders, raise shoulders toward ears and
lower them to feel the neck lengthen. Repeat and let the
head drop forward when the shoulders lift and return head
to upright position as shoulders lower.

Exercise N.   Shoulder Circles

Circle shoulders by bringing them forward, down, back,
and up. Then reverse circling by bringing them forward,
up, back, and down.

Exercise O.   Arm Extensions

Extend the right arm forward and upward slowly and then
relax it so it drops limply to side of body. Repeat with left
arm. Extend both arms forward and upward using a breath
to lift arms, then relax arms and exhale while lowering
them.

Exercise P.   Arm Exercise—"Climbing" or "Building"

Put one hand on top of the other alternately as you raise them upward (like building layers on top of one another). Then "disassemble" the building by alternately placing one hand beneath the other as you lower the arms. Try to raise the arms and hands to eye level and then return progressively to lap level.

Exercise Q.   Arm Swings

Swing one arm forward and backward letting arm hang loosely at the side. Use right arm and then left arm, then swing both arms forward and backward, gradually increasing the arc upward in front.

Exercise R.   Lateral Torso Stretch

Bend torso to the right side and slide the right arm along the side of the chair as low toward the floor as possible and then slide up. Repeat to the left side. Try to keep the head facing forward rather than downward.

Exercise S.   Upper Back and Arm Exercise

With hands clasped at the neck, bring the elbows forward. Press back with the neck as the elbows are opened out to the sides.

Exercise T.   Modified "Zipper" Stretch

Raise the right arm overhead and bend the elbow and touch the right hand to the back of the neck (as though touching the top of a zipper or a necklace). Repeat with the left arm.

Exercise U.   Upper Spine Extension (Figure 4–15)

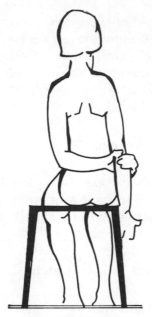

Figure 4-15   Upper spine extension. Kassoy

Extend the right arm down at side with the palm facing front. Bring the left arm behind the body and clasp the inside of the right elbow. Repeat on the other side. Try to keep the torso erect in the chair.

Exercise V.   Waist Twist

With the hands on the waist, twist from side to side, turning to look over shoulder in direction of twist. Do this four times.

Exercise W.   Leg Extension and Rotation (Figure 4–16)

Place hands under right thigh, lift knee upward and extend leg forward. Then rotate leg outward so that toes and knee face sideward. Relax leg and return to starting position.

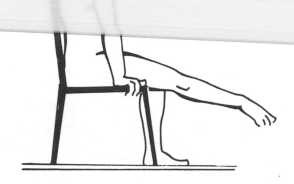

Figure 4-16   Leg extension and rotation. Kassoy

Exercise X.   Ankle Rotation

Extend one leg forward and circle the foot at the ankle in a clockwise direction and then counterclockwise direction. Repeat with the other leg.

Exercise Y.   Leg Extensions and Lifts

Extend the legs forward, lift one or both legs and place apart to the side on the floor. Lift same leg or both legs, return to closed position. Lift legs (one or both) and, in a controlled way, lower to floor, bend knee(s), bring legs to starting position. The length of time the leg is held in a raised position (near horizontal) may be increased gradually.

Exercise Z. Foot Exercise (Figure 4–17)

> Moving foot up and toward the leg.
> Moving foot down and away from the leg.

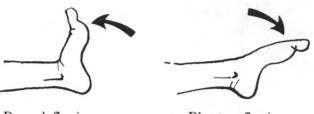

Dorsal flexion   Plantar flexion

Figure 4-17 Foot exercise. (From *Elementary Rehabilitation Nursing Care*, U. S. Public Health Service, Division of Nursing.)

Extend one leg forward, flex, and extend ankle and foot. (Toes point upward and forward.) Then bend the knee and return leg to place. Repeat with the other leg.

Exercise AA. Ankle, Arch, and Lower-Leg Exercise

Raise the heels together off the floor four times and then raise the toes of both feet off the floor four times. (Do this with feet in a vertical line below knees, while sitting.)

Exercise BB. Leg Exercise

Keep legs as close together as possible. While feet remain on floor, move legs so knees and toes face the right diagonal, then move knees and toes to face the left diagonal.

Exercise CC. Hand Massage

Using one hand to massage the other hand, gently and firmly extend and stroke each finger in turn, first one hand and then the other. Repeat.

PHYSICAL ACTIVITIES FOR THE THERAPEUTIC SESSION   99

Exercise DD.   Torso Extension with Breathing

Inhale and raise chest, then lift head slowly toward the
ceiling and return to starting position. Exhale and lower
chest, then round back and lower head. Then return to
starting position with normal breathing.

Mild Activities for the Seriously Disabled and Infirm Elderly

Programs in this category may include shortened warm-ups
with greater emphasis placed on creative work, since the
patient often is receiving physical therapy regularly. But it
is important to offer exercises that encourage increased
range of motion in order to prevent deformities. Rehabilitation for arthritic, hemiplegic, and fracture patients
should include activities to overcome limited joint flexibility (26).

Exercise A.   Hand Exercise

With elbows bent close to the body, make fist and then
relax fingers. Repeat four times.

Exercise B.   Hand-and-Arm Exercise

"Wind a Bobbin" and hammering gestures with fists and
arms, interspersed with shaking to relax.

Exercise C.   Arm-and-Torso Action

Using a slight forward and backward leaning or rocking
motion of the torso, pantomime rowing with the arms. For
one-armed action, twist slightly and imitate "poling" a raft
or paddling a canoe on one side of the body.

Exercise D.   Hand Exercise

Exaggerate the actions of hand washing—rubbing, rotating, and flexing and extending the fingers.

Exercise E.   Torso Extension

Inhale and raise chest and lift head to sit taller in the chair. Then exhale and lower chest, round back, lower head, and relax in the chair. Then return to starting position with normal breathing.

Exercise F.   Arm Rotation

Extend the arms forward and rotate them from the shoulders so that the palms face upward and then downward.

Exercise G.   Wrist Exercise

Circle wrists clockwise and counterclockwise, first with the arms hanging down at the sides and then with the elbows bent so that the hands are raised at about chest height. This may be done with one hand at a time.

Exercise H.   Eye Exercises

Look up and look down without moving the head; then blink the eyes; close and open the eyes. Do this series two times.

Exercise I.   Facial Exercises

Pantomime kissing; blow an imaginary balloon so that the cheeks are filled with air; then press the air out with hands at cheeks.

Exercise J.   Neck Massage

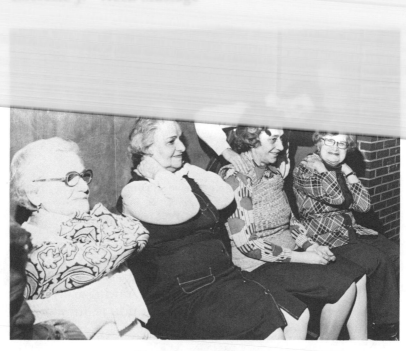

Photo 2   Neck Massage
Mike M. Miyata

With head lowered, gently massage back of neck with hands, then relax head to each side and gently stroke sides of neck.

Exercise K.   Neck Exercise

Move head in a slow, smooth sequence up toward the ceiling and down toward the floor (saying "Yes"), and then to one wall and to the other wall (saying "No").

Exercise L.   Shoulder Exercise (Figure 4–18)

Shrug shoulders up and down singly and then together.

Lifting shoulder toward the ear.
Lowering shoulder toward the hip.

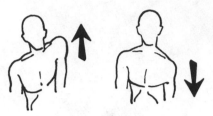

Elevation   Depression

Figure 4-18   Shoulder exercise. (From *Elementary
Rehabilitation Nursing Care,* U. S. Public Health
Service, Division of Nursing.)

Exercise M.   Arm Lifting

Lift one or both arms with a breath and exhale when lowering. Increase the height like waves (start raising arms to just
a few inches above the knees and continue to shoulder
height or above).

Exercise N.   Ladder Exercise

Climb an invisible ladder with one or both hands as high
as possible. The ladder can be in front or to the side of
person.

Exercise O.   Arm Circles

With arms hanging at the sides close to body, make circles
from the shoulder with the elbows extended. Circles can be
done outward and inward (away or toward body) and
should be slow and smooth motion.

Exercise P.   Side Stretch

Sitting with the hips level and the arms hanging down at
sides, bend torso first to one side and then to the other. Do

slowly, keeping head facing front, and return to upright
starting position.

Exercise Q.   Spinal Stretch

Relax head forward and round back toward the knees, then
slowly uncurl back up to sitting position.

Exercise R.   Shoulder Rotation

With arms hanging at sides while sitting erect, rotate the
arms from the shoulders so that the palms face outward,
then try to keep the shoulders down as the hands swing
slightly toward rear.

Exercise S.   Modified Half-Spinal Twist

Twist torso so that right shoulder faces the back and look
over it. Repeat to left side. Keep both hips level on chair
and move from waist up.

Exercise T.   Buttocks Exercise

Tense (contract) and relax (release) muscles of the seat, as
if you were making fists and letting go.

Exercise U.   Knee Lift and Leg Extension (Figure
4–19)

Clasp hands under thigh, raise knee and extend leg forward. Then slowly lower leg to the floor.

Exercise V.   Ankle Exercise (Figure 4–20)

Extend legs forward on the floor, turn the feet toward each
other by rotating the ankles, turn feet outward, then bring

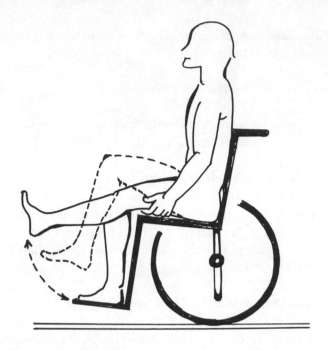

Figure 4-19   Knee lift and leg extension. Kassoy

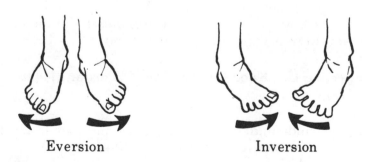

Eversion   Inversion

Figure 4-20   Ankle exercise. (From *Elementary Rehabilitation Nursing Care,* U. S. Public Health Service, Division of Nursing.)

feet back to starting position. Flex ankles so feet turn upward, extend ankles so that feet point downward.

Exercise W.   Inner Thigh Exercise

With feet together, open knees apart to the sides and then
close them together.

Exercise X.   Leg Swings

Dangle the legs (raise feet enough so they do not touch the
floor) and swing the legs forward and backward alternately
like splashing in the water.

Exercise Y.   Foot-and-Leg Exercise

With the feet on the floor, raise both heels and then lower
them. Then raise and lower the heel of each foot alternately.

Exercise Z.   Hand Exercise

Extending the arms and hands, make clawing motions like
a large catlike creature scratching a big surface.

Exercise AA.   Hand, Thigh, and Knee Massage

Rub the hands with long strokes against the top of the
thighs, first with the back of the hands and then with the
palms against the thighs. Then with firm, circling motions
cup and stroke knees.

Exercise BB.   Face Massage

Pat face gently with fingers moving quickly around from
chin to cheeks to forehead and back again, like powdering
oneself or like splashing on aftershave lotion.

Exercise CC.   Walking in Place

Lift feet alternately by raising knees and using ankle extension and flexion to simulate marching in place.

Assisted Activities for Severely Regressed, Depressed, and Disabled Patients

It is desirable to have a small group so that each patient can get individual attention. If necessary, bedridden patients may be visited in their rooms by the dance therapist. Dance/movement activities can then be conducted at the bedside.

The leader should strive to have as much physical contact as possible with each person. One begins by attempting to relate to or to comfort and then one progresses gradually to assisted activities with group members. This can be done by the therapist through eye and voice contact and then through touch. It may be possible to touch various body parts such as the shoulders and arms, for example, depending on the patient's receptivity.

Activities utilizing hand contact include subtle touching, patting, stroking, and clapping. If the patient is able to make hand contact with the leader, then gentle finger playing or "hand dancing" can be very effective to encourage the extension of the arms and the response of the torso.

The leader-therapist can sit in a chair opposite an individual and, after establishing contact (physical or visual), they may be able to rock together in a forward and backward or side to side pattern.

With the regressed or depressed clients, music is extremely helpful to raise the energy levels and to provide rhythmic impulse.

A response may be elicited by mirroring or exaggerating the actions of the patient. The leader-therapist can be

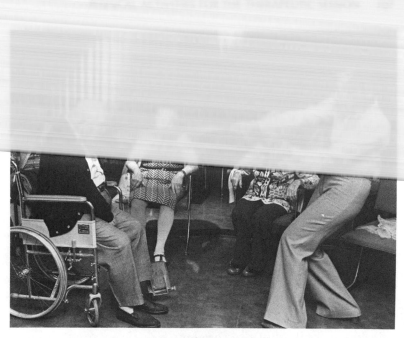

Photo 3   Therapist Working with Patient
Sam Siegel—Metropolitan Photo Service

alert to the possibility of adding to or altering a repetitive movement pattern established by the patient. For example, a person who had been habitually hitting himself in a rapid rhythm has been able to slow down that action through opportunities to use a drum in therapeutic movement sessions. He has even been able to develop an awareness of these actions and sometimes can use self-control to eliminate the motions.

It may be possible to make contact with a withdrawn person by standing or sitting at the side of the seated individual and gently leaning or rocking with him or her. Linking elbows, patting the forearm, or leaning forward and backward in time to music is often both reassuring and stimulating.

Using props such as elastic webbing in long strips, scarves, hoops, or musical instruments are often effective with this group. (See sections on "Use of Music", "Use of Props", and "Activities with Instruments".)

Some patients respond well when the therapist moves their limbs in passive activity. Many of the slow and gentle movements of the scarf sequences suggested under "Adapted Dances" can be used. Also "sharing" a scarf or a rhythm stick or bongo drums with the therapist can make participation possible. Either the therapist actually guides the action by holding the patient's hand with the object or the patient may be able to hold one end of a small scarf while the therapist holds and moves the other end.

BREATHING

A calming, quieting period, during which techniques for improved breathing and relaxation are practiced, is always offered at the end of the session's exertion. Breathing and relaxation exercises may also be interspersed between physically energetic activities throughout the session.

Values of Correct Breathing

Breathing is essential to living and the quality of living is directly influenced by the kind of breathing that is done.

The process of breathing involves the proper use of intercostal muscles, ribs, diaphragm, and abdominal muscles on the elastic capabilities of the lungs. This helps to clear the lungs of "stale" air and introduce fresh, oxygenated air to the respiratory and circulatory systems. This also helps to provide increased physical energy, mental clarity, and emotional relaxation. Gentle, rhythmic breathing has a calming effect and deep, slow breathing produces an energizing result. Caution should be taken to prevent hyperventilation, by not sustaining conscious breathing activity for long time periods.

Relationship of Breathing to Emotional States

Correct breathing is specifically related to improved posture and expanded chest, direct gaze, erect spine, and
therefore, a more positive self-image and outgoing attitude
on the part of the older person.

The mental and emotional state of the individual is
often indicated by the breathing pattern. It may reflect
agitation or withdrawal by its rapidity or shallowness. Ex-
citement, anxiety, fear, and depression are demonstrated
by variations to the normal, healthy breathing rhythm of
the individual. Here is an example from our experience.

> On the morning when a strike of hospital workers was antici-
> pated, the residents of the geriatric home were very upset.
> They were concerned over the possibility of transfers to
> other facilities and the loss of services and assistance. The
> tempo of speech and movement was faster and less con-
> trolled. There were many instances of repetitive questions
> and gestures and the concentration was poor. The dance
> therapist allowed the discussion to flow for awhile and ac-
> knowledged the participants' fears. Then she began the
> movement session with directed breathing activity. The
> group slowed down, relaxed, and tensions eased so that the
> members could focus on new ideas and activities.

Breathing Techniques

It is beneficial to introduce the older adult to the three
aspects of yoga breathing that utilize the different areas of
the lungs: low, middle, and upper. This increases awareness of the use of the respiratory mechanism and contributes to the increase of efficiency and decrease of tension.

We have found it helpful to start breathing exercise
cycles by exhaling so that one does not trap air or hyper-

ventilate. Also when working with patients who have emphysema, bronchitis, or other chronic pulmonary obstructive diseases, it may be beneficial to encourage that the exhalation be twice as long as the inhalation.

The following may be done seated in a chair with the torso upright and the feet on the floor. If the soles of the feet are pressed against the floor, the spine may respond by extending more completely.

1.   Abdominal Breathing (lower)
The hands may be placed on the upper abdomen to feel the outward and inward movement produced by diaphragm action. This promotes the greatest use of the lungs for cleansing action.

(a) "Ha." Inhale through the nostrils as the diaphragm lowers and the abdomen is pushed out. Then say "Ha" and the air is forcefully expelled from the lungs as the diaphragm rises and the abdomen is pulled in toward the spine. Three repetitions are sufficient for most groups.

(b) "Blowing Slowly." Inhale through the nose as the abdomen is pushed out, then the air is smoothly and slowly exhaled through pursed lips as the abdomen is pulled in (almost twice as slowly as the inhalation). After practice, use two counts to inhale and four counts to exhale.

(c) Slow, nasal breathing. Inhale and exhale through the nostrils rhythmically to an even, slow count of approximately three counts for each phase.

2.   Rib Cage Breathing (middle)
The diaphragm is not involved so the abdomen does not react during breathing, but remains neutral as the chest activates the inhalation and the exhalation. Place the hands at sides of ribs with fingers toward each other to feel the widening and narrowing of the chest. Slowly and evenly inhale and exhale through the nose to a rhythmic count as the middle lungs become emptied and refilled.

system. Maximum mus... benefits.

Other breathing activities to encourage relaxation and "unwinding":

4. Inhale as the arms are raised overhead, exhale as the arms are lowered.
5. With elbows bent, hands in front of chest, inhale as the arms open to the sides, then exhale as the hands return to the front of the chest.
6. While inhaling slowly, raise arms to shoulder height in front of the body, then make fists like grabbing something suddenly and lower arms quickly while forcefully exhaling through the nose.
7. The following exercises, described in the section on "Suggested Exercise Sequences," include emphasis on breathing dynamics; see pages 78, 80, 81, 82, 85, 86, and, 87, energetic exercises A, M, V, and BB, moderate exercises O, DD, and mild exercises E and M.

RELAXATION

Importance of Relaxation

The principles of consciously releasing tension need to be learned and practiced so that the effects of physical and emotional stress can be counteracted. When the body is held in the same position for long periods and when it reacts to stress or anxiety by tensing, then the muscles contract, there is a decrease of blood supply and pain may result. The pain is often transmitted from the direct source of strain to other body parts, such as from the neck and shoulders, down the torso to the buttocks or the legs. Built-up tension causes fatigue because of the needless amounts of energy expended. States such as anger and fear have a direct effect on the condition of the muscles, ligaments, and the circulatory system.

The relationship of the mind and the body is readily apparent when the conscious calming procedure of physical and mental "letting go" is practiced. Learning to release tension will help an individual overcome barriers to a restful sleep. Periods of relaxation are calming and revitalizing and, therefore, are usually offered at the conclusion of a session.

Suggestions for Conscious Relaxation

Most geriatric groups are conducted in sitting positions, therefore the following relaxation techniques may be done in chairs. However, we suggest that the leader-therapist recommend to participants that they try some of these methods in a lying position, possibly in bed. Group members who are physically agile may be encouraged to practice relaxation sequences while lying on the floor. We know that lying on the floor does present a problem for some individuals, even though it is ideal for relaxation. Many people may be resistant to the floor because of the physical discomfort of the hard surface or the difficulty of getting down or up from the low level. To others, the floor may symbolize dirt or loneliness or even entry into the subconscious and so is a threatening area. Relaxation needs to be a very gradual and voluntary process. Thus the degree of personal comfort and the feelings of security aroused will de-

RELAXATION IN BODIES AND THE BIOMECHANIC SENSES   125

terminal the success of relaxation techniques. We offer
these ideal relaxation positions with those understandings
in mind.

POSITIONS   The "Hook Lying" position is optimal for
relaxation (Figure 4-21). The back is supported fully by the
lying surface and there is no strain on the legs.

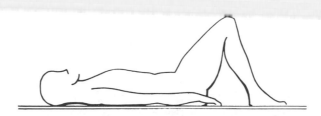

Figure 4-21   Hook lying position. Kassoy

A variation position can be lying fully extended on the
back with a small pillow placed under the knees. The arms
may be relaxed at the sides of the body or folded easily
across the chest.

Relaxation Techniques

There are two aspects to relaxation, one involving physical
activity and the other mental imagery. Ideally, an individual
will respond to both, but they can be used independently
when appropriate. In a single session, the leader-therapist
will select only one to three relaxing techniques such as the
ones we describe, preferably combining physical activity
with mental imagery. Participants are encouraged to close
their eyes while following the relaxation directions so that
concentration can be complete.

Awareness of one's body and the ability to control it
are necessary so that one can learn to relax.

The principle that uses a "rhythm of opposites" gives
one a natural way to relax because it is based on inhale-

exhale (breath), diastole-systole (heartbeat), or tense-relax (muscle action), which we all use constantly.

PHYSICAL INITIATION

1. Squeeze and Release. Tighten the muscles of various body parts for a brief period and then relax them to become aware of the ability to control and release tension. Try closing the eyes and tightening the muscles of the eyelids and face and then relax them. Repeat this with other body parts such as hands, toes, buttocks, shoulders, and so on.

2. Shaking. Shake various body parts such as hands, arms, shoulders, torso, feet, and legs. Avoid shaking the head unless initiated by the client, since it does produce dizziness in many aged persons.

3. Raising and Lowering. Raise and lower individual body parts giving in to gravity. Lift the chin up toward the ceiling and then lower the chin to the chest allowing the weight of the head to cause it to drop forward. Raise the arm just a few inches and then lower it. This may be done with the shoulders and the legs also.

4. Raising and Dropping. This may be done with the shoulders, the arms, or the knees and feet. Raise the arms a few inches and then let them fall without resisting gravity.

5. Yawning and Letting Go. Pantomime an enormous yawn using as much of the body as possible to stretch and inhale and then relax or let go.

6. Curling and Uncurling. Extend one or both arms upward, then slowly curl fingers, bend wrists, bend elbows, relax shoulders, and bring arms to sides of body. Slowly and smoothly lower head, then shoulders, then chest, and round back until torso is curled forward. Then uncurl, first the lower spine, then the chest, shoulders, and finally the head to erect posture.

7. Smoothing Face. Place palms of hands over cheeks at each side of nose, close eyes and gently slide hands

MENTAL ACTIVITIES AND THE TECHNIQUE OF RELAXA... 127

outward toward ears, smoothing face contours. Do the
same with hands placed on forehead between eyebrows and
smooth outward across brow.

IMAGERY CULTIVATION

(These images are ideally used in the back-lying position.)

1. Sand Spilling. Imagine that the body is filled with
sand. Slowly allow the sand to spill out of the legs, the
torso, the arms, and the head, through the fingertips and
the toes until you feel soft and calm.

2. Supported Weight. Let the weight of the body be
supported by the floor or the bed. Feel the body parts give
in to the support. Enjoy not resisting or working, just lying
passively.

3. Floppy Legs. Slide the feet up close to the buttocks
and then with a slight impetus let one leg at a time slide
down the floor in a floppy fashion, like a rag doll.

4. Basking in the Sun. Raise the face toward the ceiling and think about the warmth of the sun enveloping the
whole body. Try to imagine the sun's rays as they touch
each part of the body separately for a pleasurable, warm
feeling.

5. Floating Weightlessness. Visualize the body to be
so light that it is possible to feel weightless like a feather
floating.

6. Balloon or Inflated Toy. Think of the body as
though it is filled with air and then slowly let the air escape
as the body becomes softer and less tense.

7. Cool Breeze. Imagine a gentle, cool breeze moving caressingly over the body. Let it soothe and calm all
over.

8. Soothing Textures. Concentrate on textures that
are smooth or soft; these will often produce a correspond-
ing relaxation in the musculature and the mind. Images

such as silk, velvet, satin, fur, cream, and foam may be effective.

9.   Continuity Images. Thinking of repetitive or continuous movement such as circles, tides, clouds, or a gentle stream is often calming.

10.   Focus on Body Parts. Consciously direct specific parts to release tension and let go. Focus separately on the eyebrows, forehead, mouth, jaw, neck, shoulders, and so on throughout the body and "tell" each part to relax.

Caution: With each of these images there is the possibility of an individual's negative response. Therefore the leader-therapist has to be alert to the sensitivities and preferences of group members. Potentially provocative material should be presented with great care when working with geriatric clients whose emotional stability or reality orientation is insecure.

MASSAGE

Benefits of Massage in Therapeutic Movement Sessions

The most obvious benefits of massage are the improvement of circulation and the positive effects on skin and muscle tone. It also has psychological and emotional advantages such as increased self-esteem, more accurate body image, and lowered anxiety levels. Self-massage promotes a soothing and calming effect within the individual; while massage done by the leader-therapist with the client often produces feelings of reassurance and acceptance. In addition, it fosters a better interpersonal relationship because it is an opportunity to give and receive pleasurable sensations. Massage is also an excellent method of reality testing since the client recognizes him/herself and his/her place in space.

PHYSICAL ACTIVITIES FOR THE IMPAIRED AGING   117

The leader-therapist tries to reach as many individuals as possible during the dance/movement session. However, the majority of the massage activities presented in a group setting are self-massage. There are positive results to be gained by each person doing his/her own massage. Through our experiences we have found that the touching involved in the massage produces immediate positive response in almost all aged persons, especially if their physi-cal activities are limited and they are often confined to a wheelchair or bed.

Suggestions for Geriatric Massage

The kinds of massage that are used most effectively with the elderly are: stroking (*effleurage*), gentle kneading (*pétressage*), and quick, light fingertip tapping (*tapotement*). We believe that stroking and gentle kneading are more appropriate than deep massage such as the Rolfing, Swedish, or Hoffa techniques. Massage motions used on the arms and legs are done primarily toward the heart. The client is fully clothed and is usually seated. Only those areas of the body that are easily accessible, free of orthopedic appliances, and without handicapping conditions can be massaged during the dance/movement sessions.

Massage Techniques

The primary areas that are massaged during a therapeutic dance/movement session are the arms, face, hands, neck, spine, thighs, and knees.

1. Arm Massage. Knead the upper arm like squeezing dough and stroke the entire arm with long, smooth motions from wrist to shoulder. Use gentle, circular motions around the elbow.

2.   Face Massage. Using both hands simultaneously, the face can be patted or tapped with the fingertips or the palms in upward and outward directions.

3.   Back-and-Spine Massage. Stroke the back by moving both hands strongly upward and outward on either side of the spine from the waist toward the shoulders. Then, starting below the waist level, if possible, move the thumbs up the spine, one over the other, with gentle pressure toward the head.

4.   Thigh-and-Knee Massage. Use gentle, circular motions on the knee cap and upward stroking action behind the knee. Gently tap the top, bottom, and sides of the thighs.

5.   The following exercises, described in the section on "Suggested Exercise Sequences," involve additional massage techniques; see pages 81, 98, 100, 101, 105, energetic exercise I, moderate exercise CC, and mild exercises, D, J, AA, and BB.

6.   The relaxation technique on page 113 utilizes massage action.

DANCE/MOVEMENT SESSION

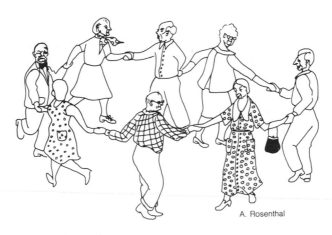

A. Rosenthal

Creative Expression

The Importance of Expressive and Creative Activities

The characteristic commonly found among older adults is the sense of isolation. Thus, participation in group activities that provide outlets for positive and negative emotions in an accepting and encouraging atmosphere, develops the individual's sense of community. We believe in the statement, "in dancing with you, I accept you." Movement sessions enable people to establish a more meaningful relationship with others. The expressive and creative activities form an extremely important part of the dance/movement program because they are necessarily nonpressured, playful, and socializing in nature. They provide participants with the opportunity to express themselves as people rather than as patients. The institutionalized elderly often have additional difficulties such as lack of reality contact, disorientation in relation to time, person, or place, extreme mood swings, and severe withdrawal. The dance therapist provides reality orientation through basic information given repetitiously and facts continuously reinforced. Also the leader remotivates by stimulating sensory awareness and establishing new neural patterns.

A complete therapeutic movement program will include activities that are structured and comparatively formal plus those that are more improvisational and freely developed by the client.

The range of creative activities available to the dance therapist is extensive and utilizes sources such as dance, drama, music, mime, and games. This variety of source material makes it possible to encourage responsiveness from participants even though they may be limited physically, emotionally, or socially. Expressive and creative activities are an excellent way of establishing a sense of personal identity and developing one's inner resources. Modern dance is used most frequently when free expression or physical interpretation is desired. The unlimited, natural use of the body can then be encouraged without restricting the individual to a learned vocabulary of movements. When the security of familiar steps and patterns are a welcome introduction to personal response, then folk dance has proved to be an ideal medium. The simple, repetitive patterns offer safety and ritual power. Many ethnic forms use the circle which encourages group solidarity. Most authentic music for folk dancing is well accented and brings a style or flavor to the session. This may evoke a desired mood or expression of joy, peace or strength. Other values of using folk dances are the necessary interde-

position of hand or shoulder contact, the reaching up and out gestures, and the sense of personal identity developed through ethnic and cultural themes.

Cautions for the Use of Free Expression

Many older adults respond to creative activities such as dance and rhythmic movement with eagerness and delight. But for some, there are disturbing or threatening elements inherent in free expression. The leader-therapist needs to be aware of the following potential problems that may exist for certain clients.

The playful quality of rhythmic activity may seem childish for the elderly who have been treated in patronizing ways or who are insecure about their maturity or competence. Some clients may also have a lack of play experiences in their backgrounds, and this delightful method of self-expression will have to be introduced gradually and gently. Many older people may have strong feelings of deprivation and rejection to work through and so need a great deal of supportive help.

Unexpected or unusual elements may be frightening or discomforting for someone who is fiercely clinging to minimal signs of stability in a rapidly changing life.

Free movement, or the invitation to let oneself be carried by the music so that new dimensions or feelings may be revealed, can be threatening. Some people cannot risk releasing violent or unconscious feelings that they feel they may not be able to control.

Motions using body parts in ways that are associated with flirtation, seduction, or physical pleasure may be viewed as "sexy" or vulgar.

Competitive challenge evoked by watching others participate or by noting the reactions of the leader to other group members may be too difficult to handle. For some who have always functioned in a competitive situation, the absence of specific goals or definite recognition may be unsatisfying.

The reassuring, low-keyed, nonjudgmental attitude of the leader-therapist helps most group members to overcome these blocks to self-expression. The leader provides limits to keep the patients from being overwhelmed by directing the movements or by structuring the rhythmic form. Suggestions such as using different body parts to express anger or violence (elbows, head, hips, or feet) or experimenting with varieties of energies (punching, stroking, slashing, tickling, flailing, patting, pushing, jabbing) can help focus on the individual's ability to "let go" and still retain control and the power of choice.

Other aids for the client's ease in self-expression include the un-self-conscious participation of the leader in whatever is suggested for the group. Also the emphasis on the activity and the importance of fulfilling one's own goals, rather than concern for performance or the reactions of others will reduce anxiety.

Values of Adapted Dance Patterns

Most dance patterns are overly vigorous or too complicated for the aged. There are some instructions for square and folk dances that are simple enough to be used effectively for active groups of well elderly. But the alteration of well-known folk, jazz, and social dances or the creation of new movement sequences will provide dance patterns that are more suitable for the general geriatric population.

Adapted dance patterns offer a geriatric group opportunities for positive recall through the use of familiar melodies and also provide memory stimulation through the repetition of sequences. Other reasons for including dances in the expressive part of the therapeutic session are the benefits of improved coordination, body awareness, self image, and the sense of accomplishment that they offer. The fulfilled challenge of remembering a series of actions and the ability to perform them within a rhythmic structure gives an important sense of accomplishment and group solidarity.

Guidelines for Adapting Dance for the Elderly

The choice of simple dances does not imply selecting child-like or coy activities that would be demeaning or embarrassing for older adults. Many senior citizens are selective, sophisticated people with years of fruitful experiences to draw on. They will appreciate respect for their maturity in the form of pleasant, strongly rhythmic, uncomplicated dance patterns. The most suitable movement sequences are those that are easily executed because they are simple, physically undemanding, and comfortably fitted to the musical phrasing. It is also helpful if they are brief enough to be repeated and enjoyed a few times in one session. Often, traditional dances can be modified by changing the emphasis on footwork to torso or arm movements. One may reduce to a minimum the number of different patterns that can then be repeated with only slight variations. To make partner dances more appropriate, they can be rearranged for single participants. Dances that are presented for couples should require limited interaction and responsibility for someone else. When assistants and/or volunteers are available, they are desirable as partners.

In order to provide a variety of style and energy use for geriatric groups, the leader-therapist can make selections for adapted dance patterns from many ethnic sources. For example, the gentle, flowing movements of Viennese waltzes, the vigorous and controlled motions of Slavic work dances, and the delicate and precise actions of Oriental dances can be found in many different cultures. Israeli and Serbian dances can provide rocking, leaning, and close body contact with shaking or clapping movements. African and Latin dances often have strongly accented motions of the feet, arms, or pelvis.

Instructions for Nineteen Adapted Dance Patterns

The following are our original adaptations of traditional dance patterns that we have used successfully with diverse geriatric groups. Each dance is outlined in two versions: Group I—Standing, for ambulatory or active adults, and Groups II and III—Sitting, for physically limited or disabled persons. The instructions are helpful for general structure, but the emphasis is not on perfect execution. So don't insist on specific details when leading. Directions for right and left or particular body parts should be very flexible and broad adaptations according to individual limitations or abilities should be accepted. All group members are encouraged to participate and enjoy the overall experience.

Educational Activities Record, AR85, was produced by the authors and offers especially appropriate musical accompaniment and detailed instructions for dances, exercises, and rhythm games.

1.   Row, Row, Row Your Boat—"Action Songs & Rounds," HYP508;Educational Activities Record Co.

This dance relies on the group participating in the familiar song as accompaniment for the movements. If the group is able, it may be done as a two- or four-part round in singing and in movement.

Group I—Standing

Measures:

1. "Row, row, row your boat"
Stretch arms forward and bend knees, bring arms back with hands to chest (like rowing) and straighten knees. Repeat.

2. "Gently down the stream"
Sway to right and left while lifting arm and leg on opposite side. Repeat.

3. "Merrily, merrily, merrily, merrily"
Clap hands four times as arms are lifted forward and upward. (If possible, turn completely around with four steps while clapping.)

4. "Life is but a dream"
Open arms in a circle like yawning and place both hands near one ear to mime sleeping.

Groups II and III—Sitting

1. "Row, row, row your boat"
Rock torso forward and backward twice while using arms in rowing motion.

2. "Gently down the stream"
Rock the body from side to side twice.

3. "Merrily, merrily, merrily, merrily"
(a) For those who can—swing legs like splashing in the water.
(b) Or, instead, shake hands up in the air.

4. "Life is but a dream"
Stretch arms upward and outward, making a large circle like a yawn. On the word "dream" place both hands near one ear and mime sleeping.

2. "Tea for Two"—"Special Music for Special People," AR85;Educational Activities Record Co.

Group I—Standing

Measures:

1. Touch right foot to right side, return to place. Repeat.
2. Touch left foot to left side, return to place. Repeat.
3. Clap hands and tap right foot with right hand.
4. Repeat (3) on left side.
5. Push right hand forward four times while turning right in complete circle.
6. Repeat (5) with left arm, while turning left.
7. Circle right arm and then left arm while bouncing with knees.
8. Circle both arms outward slowly while raising head.

Groups II and III—Sitting

Dance is the same as the standing version except:

3–4. Clap hands and tap thigh instead of foot.
5–6. Do not execute a turn.
7. Circle each arm without knee bounces.

3. "Hukilau"—"Special Music for Special People" AR85; Educational Activities Record Co.

This is a Hawaiian fishing dance and the hand movements are mimetic and typical of Oriental dance.

Group I—Standing

The basic foot pattern: step together, step, is used throughout, either in place or with direction as indicated.

Measures:

1. "We're going to a Hukilau"
   Two wrist circles to the right, basic step to the right side.
2. "Huki, huki, huki, huki, hukilau"
   Two wrist circles to the left, basic step to the left side.
3. "Everybody loves a hukilau"
   Hands do beckoning action in front of chest.
4. "Where the Lau Lau is the Kau Kau at the Luau"
   Spread fingers in front of eyes, make a big smile as hands open to the sides. Basic step done in place two times.
5. "Oh we throw our nets out into the sea"
   Both hands over one shoulder, make an arcing motion overhead and downward in front of body like throwing a net.
6. "And all the Ama Ama come swimming to me"
   Place one hand on top of the other and with swimming action of hands mime a fish going from one side to other.
7. Repeat (1 and 2).
8. "What a beautiful day for fishing"
   Describe a large circle with both hands going up, out, and down.
9. "The old Hawaiian way"
   Put fingertips of both hands together to make a thatched roof.
10. "And the Hukilau nets are swishing down in old Laie Bay"

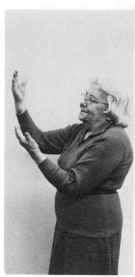
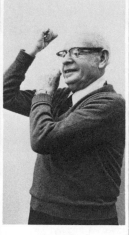
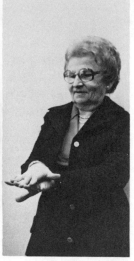
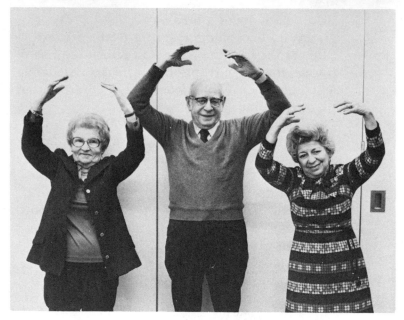

Photo 4　Hukilau
Mike M. Miyata
(a) Beckoning Gesture
(b) Holding Fishing Net
(c) Swimming Gesture
(d) Arm Circle for "What a beautiful day . . ."

Turn hands over with fingertips still touching
and do scooping motions diagonally to the right
and to the left.
11. Repeat (1–10).
12. Repeat (1–7).

Then, to complete the music phrase, do "pulling" motion twice on right side and twice on left side, then with
shaking motion bring arms overhead and extend them forward, palms down, one on top of the other and incline head
forward.

Groups II and III—Sitting

Same as standing version, without foot pattern.

4. "Anniversary Waltz"—"Special Music for Special People," AR85; Educational Activities Record Co.

This is a scarf dance. Small head scarves or handker-
chief-sized cloths may be used. Bright colors are particularly appreciated.

Group I—Standing

Circle formation, each person holding the ends of a
scarf with people on each side.

Measures:

1– 2. Walk in toward center of circle lifting arms.
3– 4. Walk backward away from center lowering arms.
5– 8. Balance to the right and to the left (rock or sway sideward).

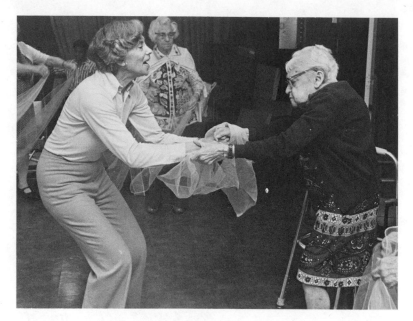

Photo 5   Anniversary Waltz—Scarf Dance
Sam Siegel—Metropolitan Photo Service

9–12.   Slowly turn alone letting scarf wave at waist or chest level.
13–16.   Walk in single circle counterclockwise holding scarves.

Repeat from beginning.

Groups II and III—Sitting

Each person holds a scarf at one end.

Measures:

1– 4.   With scarf in right hand, move arm forward and backward two times.
5– 8.   Repeat arm swinging in left side.

9–12.   Hold ends of scarf in both hands and sway
        side to side twice.
13–16. Still holding both ends, lift scarf up (if pos-
        sible over head to touch neck), and then
        down.
17–20. With scarf end in right hand, make four
        small circles.

21–24. Repeat four small circles with left hand
        holding scarf.
25–28. Repeat (9 through 12).
29–32. Still holding both scarf ends, lift scarf up
        over head and place around neck, leave it
        and place hands in lap with a clap.

**5. *"Patch Tanz"—"Israeli Folk Dance Medley," LPT
        106; Tikva Records or Folkraft
        118x45A***

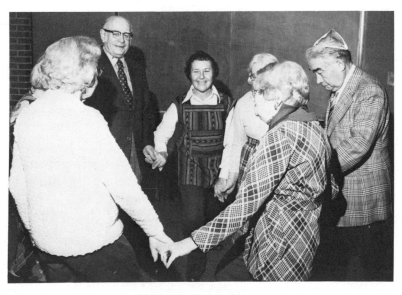

Photo 6   Patch Tanz
Mike M. Miyata

Group I—Standing

Measures:

    1– 4. Circle to the right for 16 steps.

    5– 6. Face center of circle and walk 4 steps in and clap three times.

    7– 8. Take 4 steps back out of circle and stamp three times.

    9–12. Repeat (2 and 3).

  13–16. Those who can, take a partner and turn holding with right elbows linked or both hands clasped. Without a partner, turn slowly in a complete circle alone or sway in place in time to the music.

Groups II and III—Sitting

Measures:

      1. Stretch arms forward—four counts.

      2. Put hands on hips—four counts.

    3– 4. Repeat (1 and 2).

      5. Clap three times.

      6. Stamp three times (or clap hands to thighs).

    7– 8. Repeat (5 and 6).

    9–10. With both arms together, snap fingers making a big circle from the left over head to the right side—eight counts.

  11–12. Repeat circling from the right to the left with snapping—eight counts.

6. "Cherkessia" ("Circassia")—"Special Music for Special People," AR85; Educational Activities Record Co.

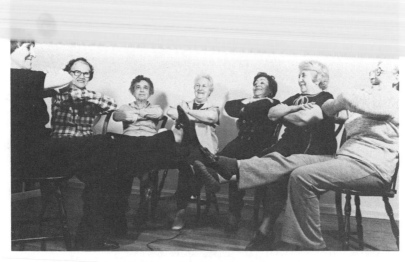

Photo 7   Cherkessia
Robert Blucher

Group I—Standing

Chorus: Take a small lunging step forward on the first beat of music and then take three small steps in place. Do this pattern four times and repeat after each new stanza.

Stanzas: On each stanza one person at a time is the leader and initiates a movement in place which everybody emulates. (They can be arm or hand movements, body gestures, and so on.)

Groups II and III—Sitting

Chorus: Clap the rhythm of the circassia step (loud, soft, soft, soft claps repeated three times).

Stanzas: Same as for Group I unless the leader-therapist finds it necessary to be the initiator for all new motions at first, and then can call for specific people to give suggestions. Sometimes work movements or familiar gestures of everyday activities can be mimed.

7. "Bingo"—"Around the World in Dance," AR542; Educational Activities Record Co. or RCA Victor EPA 4138

Group I—Standing

Group members march around the room during the first 32 counts of music. When the slow "B" is played they shake one hand of the person nearest to them; on the "I" they shake the other hand of that person; on "N" and "G" they hold both hands and shake twice; and on "O" they lift both arms overhead and let go. The music resumes and they continue to walk around until they find a new partner for the slow chorus to be repeated.

Groups II and III—Sitting

On the marching music:

Measures:

1–4. Everybody claps 16 times.
5–6. Everyone stamps their feet 8 times.
7–8. Everyone snaps their fingers 8 times.

On the slow chorus:
The leader-therapist shakes hands with one person at a time, moving around the room to a different person on each signal B-I-N-G-O so that five people are greeted before the music starts over again.

Group I—Standing

The hand-and-arm patterns are the same for sitting or standing versions. Those people able to walk or "jig" can add a rocking foot pattern in place, a side grapevine step, and a lunge step forward on alternating feet to the arm movements.

Groups II and III—Sitting

Four measures—"Hitching Trousers"—to start the sailor's voyage pull up trousers with one hand in front and one in back at waist level, alternate hands with each four counts, do four times.

Four measures—"Haul in the Anchor"—to free the ship lean forward diagonally right with hands grasping imaginary rope on one count; pull back toward body for three counts. Alternate left and right and left sides.

Four measures—"Raise the Sail"—to catch the wind, pull down an imaginary rope from overhead into lap with alternating arm on each four counts, do four times.

Four measures—"Ahoy"—look to see ahead, shade the eyes with the right hand and turn to look right; repeat with left hand to left and then do two more times.

Four measures—"Clear Sailing Ahead"—relax and roll with the waves, clasp hands in front of body with palms facing down, rock arms from side to side four times.

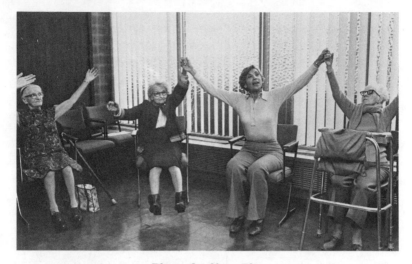

Photo 8   Shoo Fly
Sam Siegel—Metropolitan Photo Service

9. "Shoo Fly" Folkraft Records 1185

Group I—Standing

Group in single circle formation holding hands.

Measures:

1. All walk four steps to center raising hands upward.
2. Back out of circle four steps lowering hands.
3–4. Repeat (1 and 2).
5–6. Take partner next to you with two hands and walk in a circle in place together for four steps.
7–8. Change partner to person on other side and circle for four steps.

Return to single circle and start dance from beginning.

Groups II and III—Sitting

Sitting in chairs in circle or semicircle.

Measures.

1–4. Do individually with arm movements only.
5–8. Gently tap the hands of the person on either side.

10. "Seven Jumps" RCA Victor EPA 4138

A "successive" dance, in which additional motions are added with each new repetition. Chorus is performed the same way between each new and longer "stanza."

Group I—Standing

*Chorus: group members walk around the room with 16 slow steps.

Stanza: First chord—lift right arm up and lower.
          Second chord—lift left arm up and lower.

Repeat chorus from *.

Stanza: First chord—lift right arm and lower.
          Second chord—lift left arm and lower.
          Third chord—raise right leg and lower.

After each stanza repeat *, then add each successive movement in turn as additional chords are added to stanza.

          Fourth chord—raise left leg and lower.
          Fifth chord—lift chin toward ceiling and replace.
          Sixth chord—lower chin to chest and replace.

Seventh chord—raise shoulders toward ears and replace.
Eighth chord—place hands on opposite elbows across chest.

After the last stanza extend both arms up toward the ceiling for the final musical beat.

Groups II and III—Sitting

*Chorus: on the chorus clap the hands in front of the chest, alternating the right hand and then the left hand on top.
Stanzas: same as for Group I.

11.   "Mexican Waltz" "Music For Special Children," HLP 4074; Hoctor Records

Group I—Standing

Measures:

1– 3.	Swing arms from side to side three times.
4.	Clap hands two times.
5– 8.	Repeat (1–4).
9–11.	Put right heel forward, left heel forward, right heel forward.
12.	Stamp two times.
13–16.	Repeat (9–12).

For people who are able to move around, the second half of the dance may be done with a partner waltzing around the room for 16 waltz steps. (Measure 17–32)

Or:

17–18.	Swing right arm forward, backward.
19–20.	Make a circle with right arm.

21–24.   Repeat (17–20) with left arm.
25–31   Make a very slow, large circle with both
         arms.
32.   Clap hands two times.

Groups II and III—Sitting

If participants can use legs and feet, the same movements
of Group I may be done in a sitting position. If only the
arms and torso can be used then the following variation is
suggested.

Repeat (1–4) four times.
Do (17–32) as above.

12.   *"Never On Sunday" United Artists Recording,*
UA 1602 A45

During introduction, snap fingers and sway for 14
counts. If unable to snap, then clap hands.

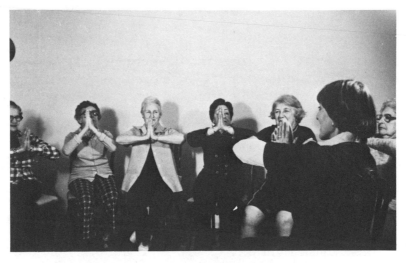

Photo 9   Never on Sunday—Measure 7
Robert Blucher

Group I—Standing

Formation: closed or open circle, holding hands at shoulder height with elbows bent.

Measure:

1. Step on right foot to the right (count 1).
   Extend left foot forward and tap it on the floor (count 2).
   Cross left foot in back of right and step on it (count 3).
   Step on right foot to the right (count "and").
   Cross left foot in front of right and step on it (count 4).
2. Step forward with right foot (1), then close left foot next to right foot (&), then step forward again with right foot (2).
   Step backward with left foot (3), then close right foot next to left foot (&), then step backward with left foot (4).

Repeat these two measures throughout music. Try lowering the arms and the head as you move toward the center of the circle and raise the arms and the head as you move backward out from the center of the circle.

Groups II and III—Sitting

Measures:

1. Touch right foot forward and bring back to place.
   Touch left foot forward and bring back to place.
2. Touch right foot to right side and bring back to place.
   Touch left foot to left side and bring back to place.

6. Push right arm out to right side while turning head to right.

4. Slowly press and lower right arm down to right side.

5. Push left arm out to left side while turning head left.

6. Slowly press and lower left arm down to left side.

7. Press both hands together and slowly raise them overhead as head lifts.

8. Open arms sideward and press down to sides.

13. *"Easy Winners" "Special Music for Special People," AR85; Educational Activities Record Co.*

This is an adapted version of the soft-shoe cane dance. Participants may hold short wands, sticks or canes.

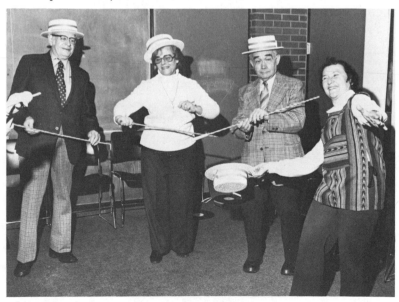

Photo 10   Easy Winners
Mike M. Miyata

Group I—Standing

Measures:

1. Turn right foot outward and extend arm with cane sideward. Return to place.
2. Repeat (1).
3. Extend right heel forward on floor and touch cane to right shoulder. Return to place.
4. Repeat (3) with left heel and touch left shoulder.

5–8. Repeat (1 through 4).

9. With cane in both hands, extend arms forward, bend knees, lean forward. Return to place.
10. Bend knees and lift head as arms extend upward. Return to place.
11. Step forward: right, close, right and left, close, left while holding cane at chest level with slight torso twist.
12. Repeat (11) moving backward.

13–16. Repeat (9–12).

17. Lift right knee touching cane to knee, replace.
18. Repeat with left knee.
19. Lunge to right side with right leg while extending right arm holding cane to right side. Return to place.
20. Repeat (19) on left side.
21. Hold top of cane with both hands and tap cane on floor as you tap right foot to side, tap cane again as you close right foot to left.
22. Repeat two taps of cane on floor in front as left foot opens side and then closes.

23–24. Twirl cane with two hands in front of chest while marking time in place with feet.

CREATIVE ACTIVITIES   143

Groups II and III—Sitting

Same pattern with exception of walking, knee bending,
and lunging action in (9–12) and (19 and 20).

14.   "Consider Yourself At Home" "Special Music For
Special People,"
AR03, Educational

*Activities Record
Co.*

This is excellent for socializing and rhythmic stimulation.

Group I—Standing

For ambulatory groups this is a "progressive" activity
in which more people join in with each repetition.

Measures:

1–4.   Leader or one person chosen from group
walks around the other waiting members
16 steps while they clap 16 times.

5–8.   Walking person stops in front of someone
and shakes right hands—four counts; left
hands—four counts; both hands—four
counts; and then helps them to stand or
join the walking path.

Now two people repeat (1–4) and then each chooses another person to shake hands with and invite to join in the
walk around. Then there will be four people doing the
walking phrase and this progression continues until everyone who can is selected to walk around the room at the
same time.

Group II—Combination of Sitting and Standing

When there are some group members who are more active than others, half of the group can remain sitting while the rest can do the ambulatory activity.

"A" (those able to march) form a circle in back of "B" (those people seated in chairs).

Measures:

1–4. "A" marches counterclockwise for 16 counts while "B" claps.

5–7. "A" walks into circle facing "B" and shakes hands for 12 counts.

8. "A" walks in back of "B" and places hands on "B's" shoulders for 4 counts.

Repeat from (1) choosing different partners each time, if possible.

(This can be done with leader-therapist and assistants or volunteers doing "A" and group members taking "B" part.)

Group III—Sitting

Group sitting in circle formation.

Measures:

1–4. Everyone claps 16 counts. (Variations: finger snapping, foot tapping, clapping thighs, and so on.)

5. First person shakes hands with person on the right and says: "I'm   (name)   " four counts.

6. That person in turn shakes hands with person on his/her right and says: "I'm (name)   " four counts.

Continue around circle with two more people shaking
hands and introducing themselves for eight counts (measures 7–8).

Repeat from beginning with variations. Measures 5–6
can be done clockwise and counterclockwise so that different couples relate to each other.

15.   "The Hokey Pokey"—Hoctor Records 1606 or Starline 6026

Group I—Standing

Do the original version.

Groups II and III—Sitting

Do the original version with the following variations:

Stanzas for body parts:
   Right hip: put right hand on right hip, take it off, put
right hand on right hip and rub it.
   Left hip: repeat above variation using left hand on
left hip.
   Whole self: bring your shoulders up and down, give
yourself a hug, then shake yourself.
   Backside: twist the torso to the right, to the left, to
the right and shake your shoulders.

Chorus between each body part stanza is:
   "Do the hokey pokey"—Move hands to the right and
left.
   "And you turn yourself around"—Roll your fore-
arms like the "wind-a-bobbin" gesture.
   "That's what it's all about"—Slowly clap hands
three times.

The final chorus is:
"Do the hokey pokey"—three times. Shake arms up, down and up.
"That's what it's all about"—Slowly clap hands three times.

The following dances have been adapted specifically for nonambulatory patients, consisting of small groups between 6 and 12 people. A large unobstructed space and several assistants are necessary. Initially a distance of two wheelchairs or one adult crutch length should be provided between dancers.

16.   "Oh, Susanna"—"Simplified Folk Dance Favorites," EA602; Educational Activities Record Co.

This is a wheelchair square dance
Sitting—eight people in square dance formation, facing center.

First Verse

Measures:

1.   Shake partner's right hand.
2.   Shake partner's left hand.
3–4.   Repeat (1 and 2) with your corner.*

Chorus

1.   Everybody holds hands and rocks to the right and left.

*Corner = person next to you who is *not* your partner.
Partner = person next to you in your "couple."

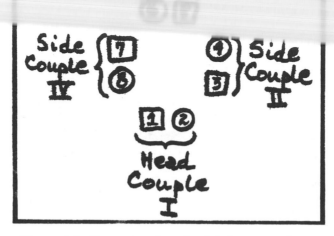

**Figure 5-1   Formation for wheelchair square dance
(People numbered counterclockwise.)**

2. Repeat (1).
3. Lift arms up and down.
4. Repeat (3).

Second Verse

1. Head couple clap hands four times.
2. Side couple repeat (1).
3. Everybody claps each other's hands sideways four times.
4. Everybody claps own hands four times.

Chorus—Repeat (1–4).

Third Verse

    1. Couple I leans forward and straightens up (one measure).

2–4. Couples No. II, III, and IV repeat (1).

Chorus—Repeat (1–4).

17. "The Man on the Flying Trapeze"—"Special Music for Special People," AR 85; Educational Activities Record Co.

    This is a wheelchair circle dance. It can be done with hand-operated wheelchairs or with gurneys.

    Sitting—Participants numbered 1 and 2 in a large single circle (Figure 5–2).

Measures:

    1– 4. Individuals move around the circle counterclockwise.

    5– 6. Go forward into the circle.

    7– 8. Back out of the circle.

    9–12. Move clockwise around the circle.

13–16. Repeat (5–8) (pause).

17–24. Face partner and turn clockwise around each other until back in place.

25–32. Turn to face your corner and repeat (17–24) counterclockwise (pause).

33–40. Move around simultaneously in two circles, No. 1 clockwise (inside), No. 2 counterclockwise (outside).

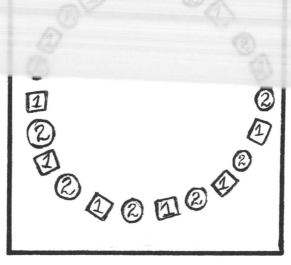

Figure 5-2 Formation for wheelchair circle dance (People numbered by "twos.")

41–44. No. 1 backs out of circle, as No. 2 goes forward into circle.

45–48. Reverse with No. 1 going forward into circle and No. 2 backs out of circle (pause).

49–52. No. 1 turns alone in place while No. 2 claps hands four times.

53–56. No. 2 turns alone in place while No. 1 claps hands four times.

57–62. Move around simultaneously in two circles. No. 1 goes clockwise (inside) and No. 2 goes counterclockwise (outside).

63–64. Face new partner. Then make a single circle, No. 1 in front of No. 2, all facing counterclockwise.

18.   "Skip to My Lou"—Folkraft 1103

This is a wheelchair square dance.
Sitting—four couples seated in a square formation facing the center.

Measures:

1. Shake hands with partner.
2. Shake hands with corner.
3. All join hands with adjacent persons and sway right and left.
4. All clap hands four times.
5. Couples I and III reach across the square and tap right hands two times with the person sitting opposite.
6. Couples II and IV repeat (5).
7– 8. Repeat (3 and 4).
9. Everyone reaches right arms upward diagonally to form a right-hand star.
10. Everyone reaches left arms upward diagonally to form a left-handed star.
11–12. Repeat (3 and 4).
13. Head couples I & III lean forward toward opposites and then sit back.
14. Side couples II and IV repeat (13).
15–16. Repeat (3 and 4).

19.   "Zemer Atik"—Worldtone WT 10007

Formation: closed circle, holding hands.

COMMUNITY AND CREATIVE ACTIVITIES   163

Group I—Standing

Measures:

1. Four walking steps counterclockwise (right, left, right, left).
2. Release hands and step on right foot, then bend right knee as you clap hands at shoulder height.

der height.
Step left and bend left knee as you clap hands at shoulder height.

3–8. Repeat (1 and 2) three more times.
9. Face center and sway right and left while waving arms from right to left overhead (with or without snapping fingers).
10. In four counts, extend the arms foward and downward as torso bends forward.
11–16. Repeat (9 and 10) three more times.

Groups II and III—Sitting

If participants can use legs and feet, the same movements of Group I may be done in a sitting position. If only the arms and torso can be used then,

Measures:

1. Tap hands against thighs four times.
2. Lean torso to right side, then clap hands near right shoulder, lean to left side and clap hands near left shoulder.
3–8. Repeat (1 and 2) three more times.
9. Twist torso to right side, then snap fingers. Twist torso to left side, snap fingers.

10. Face center, raise arms above head and slowly lower them to lap in four counts.

11–16. Repeat (9 and 10) three more times.

Other Suggestions for Adapted Dances

A comprehensive book of simple folk dances is a good resource for the dance/movement program (27). The following is a list of simple folk dances that are easily available and can be adapted by a leader-therapist for geriatric groups.

Salty Dog Rag	Korobushka	Alley Cat
Bannielou	Masquerade	Alexandrovsky
Mayim	Ve David	Boi Tama
Stack of Barley	Jessie Polka	La Raspa
Zorba	Ten Pretty Girls	Montego Bay
Tanko Bushi	Tarantella	Virginia Reel
Tante Hessie	Donegal Round	Apat, Apat
Greensleeves	Blue Tango	Pattycake Polka
Trgnala Rumjana	Karagouna	St. Bernard's Waltz

There are also many familiar tunes that may be used by the leader-therapist to arrange original step or movement sequences for simple patterns. Tunes are selected by looking for a simple melody, clear rhythmic structure, and themes that inspire action and pleasant memories. The melodies listed below can be found in collections of folk or popular music.

"Little Grass Shack"	"Harrigan"
"Goin' Dance All Over God's Heaven"	
"My Blue Heaven"	"Can Can Galop"
"Bie Mir Bist Du Schon"	"Tie A Yellow Ribbon"
	"Bicycle Built For Two"

Ballgame"   "Japanese Sandman"
"Hi Li Li"   "Matchmaker,
                               Matchmaker"
"East Side, West Side"   "Down By The Old Mill
                               Stream"
"Raindrops Keep Falling
  On My Head"   "Thoroughly Modern
                               Millie"

"Winchester Cathedral"   "When the Saints Go
                               Marching In"

"Swing Low, Sweet
  Chariot"   "The Band Played On"
"The Entertainer"   "Sunrise, Sunset"
"Happy Talk"   "Irish Washerwoman"
"Twelfth Street Rag"   "Popcorn"
"I'm Forever Blowing
  Bubbles"   "Anvil Chorus"
"Pop Goes the Weasel"   "Hava Nagila"
"Merry Widow Waltz"   "Skater's Waltz"
"Turkey In The Straw"   "Happy Days Are Here
                               Again"
"Windmuller"   "K-K-Katy"
"For Me and My Gal"   "Santa Lucia"
"La Cucaracha"   "The Happy Wanderer"
"When You're Smiling"   "Alexander's Ragtime Band"
"Funiculi Funicula"   "Happy Days Are Here
                               Again"
"Shalom Aleichem"   "You Are My Sunshine"
"Hernando's Hideaway"   "Syncopated Clock"
"Seventy Six Trombones"   "Java"

Mimetic Action Plays

The use of mime with the elderly helps to improve their
concentration, observation, and accurate responses to

ideas. Space disorientation and agnosia (unawareness of body parts) can be alleviated by simple, repetitive singing games. Such action songs as the "Hokey Pokey" stress the existence and position of body parts. Original action plays can also be created to familiar songs. Ruth Bright, a music therapist, suggests an action song to the tune of "There is a Tavern in the Town":

"Head, shoulders, knees, and toes, knees and toes,
Head, shoulders, knees, and toes, knees and toes and
Eyes and ears and mouth and nose,
Head, shoulders, knees, and toes, knees and toes."

She suggests that it can be done standing or sitting, and the group members may touch each body part named or can even look and point at them while singing the appropriate words (28).

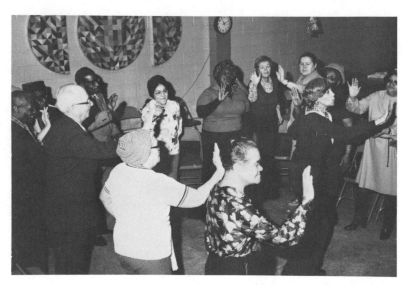

Photo 11   Dramatic Pantomime
Benjamin B. Scherman

By their inducing a number of imaginative reactions, such as dances involving dramatic pantomime elements that make them particularly suitable for group action. Many Oriental folk dances are composed of simple arm and hand movements that tell a story and provide good exercise, coordination improvement, and an ethnic experience. "Tanko Bushi" (Folkraft Records, MV 1) is a Japanese dance with coal mining gestures and a delightful rhythmic form. Other examples of this type of dance are "Hukilau" (see page 126), the Korean Tea Leaf Dance, The Canadian Logger Dance (Educational Activities Recording, EA22), and the Hawaiian "Little Grass Shack." The gesture language of Hindu dance has been used successfully to create a story that provides avenues for self-expression and release of emotional tension. Mabel Merritt, dance therapist of the Elm Hill Nursing Home in Massachusetts, writes of her group dancing a "Hindu Gesture Dance" that includes hunting and fishing movements (29). The dance leader-therapist can also arrange finger action from those suggested by the words in songs like "Happy Talk" from the musical play, "South Pacific."

The tune of "The Battle Hymn of the Republic" has been used as the basis for a few parodies that involve hand gestures and can be performed as a game of decreasing singing and increasing action. One version is "Little Peter Rabbit" and another is "John Brown's Baby." In the rabbit variation, the participants mime ears with their hands on top of their heads while singing "Little Peter *Rabbit,*" then with first finger and thumb together they gesture like a flying insect for "had a *fly,*" and then they touch their ears while singing "upon his *ear.*" These three gestures and singing phrases are repeated two more times and then as they sing "so he *wiggled,*" the group members wiggle their torsos "till it flew *away*" and then gesture with both arms at shoulder height with flying motions. This stanza is repeated but the words "Rabbit," "fly," "ear," "wiggled," and "flew" are not sung, instead they are just indicated by the gestures. The other version of "The Battle Hymn of the Republic" called, "John Brown's Baby," is especially pleasing for older people since they are reminded of children and grandchildren as babies. The song with the mimed words is "John Brown's *Baby*" (rock arms), "had a *cold*" (cough) "upon its *chest*" (tap chest) "and they *rubbed*" (make large circles on chest) "it in with *camphorated*" (hold nose with two fingers) "oil." The reminiscences of smelly camphorated oil and other home remedies adds to the enjoyment of the rhythmic action. Many warm remembrances of home and child raising have been stimulated through this mimetic activity.

The use of Biblical passages or psalms, such as the Twenty-third Psalm from the Old Testament (The Lord's Prayer), and inspiring songs like "He's Got The Whole World in His Hands" can be used for rhythmic responsive gesture. Many groups have found this a unifying experience that brings spiritual rewards.

Use of Music for Free Expression and Channeled Response

Dance is a synthesizing art form which brings together the elements of musical rhythm, dramatic expression, spatial design, and physical dynamics. Marian Chace, regarded as the pioneer and foremost leader in the field of dance therapy, used music to structure or shape her sessions and to reflect or guide the emotional tones of the group. Music and movement help the elderly to let go and again get in touch with their bodies in an appreciative manner. It can be very satisfying for an older person to recognize a melody or rhythm and respond to it physically. If the movement sequences are composed cooperatively or include favorite motions or music they become very personal means of expression. Not only do they increase the range of movement, but they serve also as an emotional outlet and can lead to social enjoyment. A good example of this aspect of music is found in the following anecdote.

Mrs. M is a handsome woman whose speech is limited by a brain lesion. She rarely utters a word but she imitates every gesture that the therapist makes. Her movements are extremely rhythmic and musical. When she stands up to dance she is beautiful to look at — graceful and totally involved. At the beginning of many sessions she is crying. As soon as the music begins, she smiles and joins the activity. She seems free and joyous during the whole dance session.

Music may evoke past experiences. The use of tunes from the 1920s and 1930s plus popular melodies and show songs are particularly effective. These reminiscences can be the intellectual stimulation that develops into therapeutic

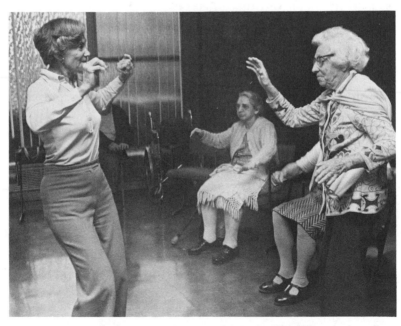

Photo 12   Music for Free Expression
Sam Siegel—Metropolitan Photo Service

discussion in addition to provoking physical activity. The motivating force of music is demonstrated by music therapist, Ruth Bright, who said, "It is not uncommon to see a patient, thought to be virtually chairbound despite the best efforts of the nursing staff, get up and waltz around the room when music which 'takes the fancy' is played" (30).

Music is also a powerful mood modifier. There are different qualities in music, such as those that are calming and soothing and others that are stimulating. The leader-therapist may choose gay and lively music or select dramatic and inspiring compositions in order to encourage reactions by the group members. It has been found by music therapist, Ruth Boxberger that . . . "less aggressiveness is exhibited by patients in nursing homes where music is used in social settings" (31).

The predetermined structure of the musical piece may be extremely helpful in channeling a desired response, or it may present problems by limiting complete freedom of expression. The length and the phrasing of the composition should be carefully considered in selecting accompaniment or inspiration.

In addition, music and instruments played for a geriatric group should be modulated at a low volume since the aged have a low tolerance for loud sounds.

There are many individuals within groups of well, active senior citizens who enjoy dancing alone or with a partner to familiar tunes. They recall steps they used on happy occasions in their younger days. Waltzes, polkas, the Peabody, and the foxtrot inspire independent activity across the dance floor. Even in homes or hospitals for the aged, there may be one or two people who are able to enjoy dancing alone or with the assistance of the leader. Gentle and careful attention must be given to the problems of balance or fatigue that might develop. The opportunity to

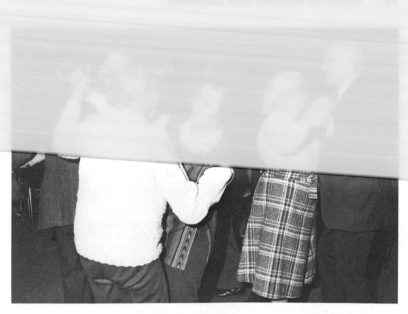

Photo 13   Social Dancing
Mike M. Miyata

dance with someone else in a close relationship is very beneficial because it provides supportive, physical contact and is a rewarding and pleasant experience. A person is aware of being accepted and enjoys being part of a couple. We can share an experience from our logs to illustrate this:

> I noticed a new woman sitting apart from the group. I invited her to move in a little closer and join us. She declined, saying she didn't feel well. After the session began, I noticed that she finally started to participate. Then I put on a tango, "Orchids in the Moonlight" and I approached her. She stood up, and we began to dance. She smiled and seemed to enjoy herself. After the session ended she said, "You made my day. I didn't sleep all last night. I was so restless and alone and anxious. Yesterday I was told that I have to have a very serious operation. You held me. And now I feel better. I feel new courage. There is a smoothness inside me.

In order to initiate original creative response to musical accompaniment, we have found these methods to be particularly successful:

1.   Play a piece of music and begin with one movement suggested by the leader and then add appropriate actions suggested by members of the group. (This is usually done without words.)

2.   As the music is playing invite everyone to respond as he/she wishes. Within a circular formation, the leader can select one appropriate movement and then another one for short periods while the group members follow or do whatever they want.

3.   Play a piece of music and encourage free improvisation by members of the group. The leader can, after the music is completed, select actions that were performed by participants and combine them to form a pattern that fits the music. The group can then perform this pattern to a repetition of the music.

4.   Play a musical selection and discuss "what it sounds like," "what it reminds one of," or "how one could move to it." Then have one half the group try moving to the music and then the other half and finally encourage everyone to join in.

A varied collection of music from which to select is an asset for a creative movement program. It helps to be able to plan several possible music choices and idea suggestions so that the spontaneous needs of the group can be met. Choral works, orchestral compositions, and pieces by small instrumental groups represent a good range. Composers such as Debussy, Brahms, Bach, Mozart, Bartok, Arthur Benjamin, Handel, Ravel, Satie, Vivaldi, Schubert, and Strauss should be included, as well as popular and nostalgic preferences. (See pages 152, 153, 223, 224, 229, 230, and 231 for specific suggestions of music.)

EXERCISE AND CREATIVE ACTIVITIES   173

Use of Objects for Socialization, Personal Expression, and Physical Mobility

The geriatric dance therapist will find that inventive and creative uses of inexpensive, easily accessible objects are great additions to the program. A good imagination uncovers delightful possibilities for old hats, scraps of fabric, and discarded paper and plastic articles. Objects that are light-weight and comfortable to manipulate provide the interest and challenge that may be necessary for improved coordination and mobility. Vivid colors and designs (use of flowers, crepe paper, contact paper, etc.) add to the attractiveness and enjoyment of the objects used. They can provide the bright spot in an old person's day. They may even inspire unexpected responses that have been long repressed. (See page 232 for list of suggested objects for a therapeutic session.)

Sharing props may foster the kind of interdependence that is often an important step toward resocialization with the lonely or regressed elderly. An example of this is the responsibility involved when holding a hoop or a scarf with someone else. A valuable technique for encouraging interaction is the use of a circle formation in which people can share and pass objects or make physical contact with each other. We have used a long length of rope (clothesline or jumprope variety) for everyone to hold. This can provide a symbolic bond or a very real aid for balance and guidance. With easy swinging or reaching movements, the whole group can move together in "joined" action.

Many design forms can be created cooperatively by using *soft armature wire,* or circles of string or elastic. With a small group of people to manipulate the material, with or without music for inspiration, shapes can be produced that may be abstract or specific. The participants should be arranged in small groups facing each other. Everyone holds onto and manipulates the wire, string, or elastic by moving

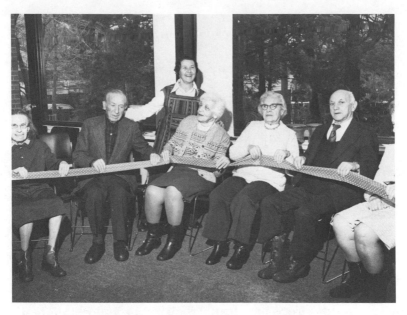

Photo 14   Group Action with Prop
Mike M. Miyata

it up and down and in and out to produce design shapes. The armature wire will remain in the shape that is produced by the group and can be preserved like a "sculpture." The *string or elastic* will result in a "line drawing," which can be seen if it is held still by the group members on a signal from the leader to stop the action and show the shape produced. It is pleasant to try this activity with group members holding a large *loop of elastic.* They move and stretch it until the music stops and they "freeze" so that everyone can admire the design formed. This can be repeated at regular or irregular musical intervals. If the group members have experimented with making string pictures with nails or tacks or have seen mobiles, they may find this a satisfying challenge for cooperative expression.

A long length (four yards or so) of *elastic webbing* such as that used for waistbands of pajamas or undershorts can

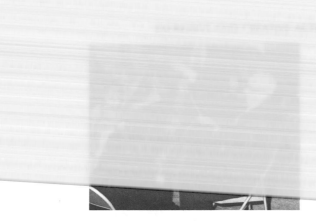

Photo 15 Line Drawing
Benjamin B. Scherman

offer many other creative movement possibilities. Arrange five or six group members in a line or a circle with each holding the elastic in one or both hands. Explore moving forward and backward, side to side, and up and down. The therapist can introduce different qualities of musical accompaniment so that stretching and pulling and twisting actions may take on different emotional tones also.

Small scarves in bright colors have unlimited potential to inspire movement ideas. Lightweight chiffon or silk squares or ribbon streamers that will float are appropriate. Easily manipulated scarves can be made by attaching a loop or an elastic to one corner of a piece of fabric. Or durable *streamers* can be produced by cutting strips 2 inches by 18 inches from a plastic trash or leaf bag. Two of these streamers can then be attached to one end of a cardboard inner roll from paper towelling or waxed paper (Figure 5–3).

1. Waltzing Activities. Hold scarf in one hand and wave it across chest and open out to the side in a figure eight motion. Wave scarf forward and upward and then downward and backward. Make full circles in front of chest or at the side or, if possible, overhead with the scarf. Repeat sequence with the other hand. Try parts of the sequence with both hands. On the chorus of the music, the group

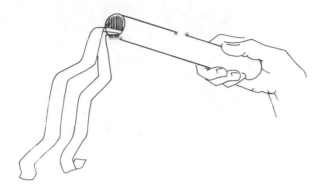

Figure 5-3   Cardboard roll with streamers. Kassoy

may be encouraged to dance with each other or stand and rock and sway to the music either alone or with someone, possibly holding the ends of each other's scarf. This might also be done sitting down with adjacent people holding their neighbor's scarf and swaying together. Waltzes that provide good accompaniment are: "Alexandrovsky," "East Side, West Side," "Anniversary Waltz," "The Band Played On," "Take Me Out To The Ball Game," "Sunrise, Sunset," and "Matchmaker, Matchmaker."

2.   Mimetic Activities. The many events of a circus suggest various ways to use a scarf rhythmically. To the tune of "The Man On The Flying Trapeze" (AR85; Educational Activities Record Co.) we have mimed the actions of a juggler (tossing and catching the scarf), a trapeze swinging, a snake charmer (with a slithering scarf), a magician (curl and release scarf from hands), an animal trainer (crack the "whip"), and a parade (wave the banner). This flag or banner waving makes a nice chorus with different "acts" for each stanza of the song.

3.   Semaphore Alphabet. Using scarves as is or attaching them to small dowel sticks, each person can learn to signal the "grand circle" of letters from A through G (Figure 5–4). If there is a group member who was in the naval service or remembers signalling from scouting or

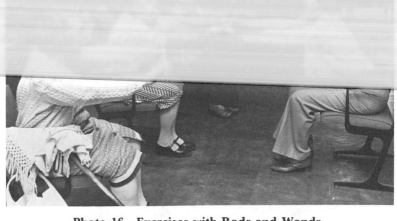

Photo 16   Exercises with Rods and Wands
Sam Siegel—Metropolitan Photo Service

railroading, it may be possible to spell words while enjoying rhythmic activity which is highly beneficial to the upper torso, in addition to the intellectual stimulation.

4.   Pantomime with Streamers. Using the cardboard rolls with plastic streamers attached (see page 164) individuals can move them in large gestures to simulate the action of riding whips, fishing poles, flags waving, baseball bats swinging, golf clubs, tennis rackets, canoe paddles, and rowing oars. The streamers can be used to describe the arc of a rainbow, the lines in a painted mural, or the motions of mixing, stirring, and decorating a cake.

We have found that inexpensive paper and wooden folding fans make delightful props for creative movement. Even folded paper or other handmade fans that can be easily manipulated work well for activities accompanied by music such as "Tit Willow" (from *The Mikado*), "Japanese Sandman," and "Happy Talk" (from *South Pacific*). Sug-

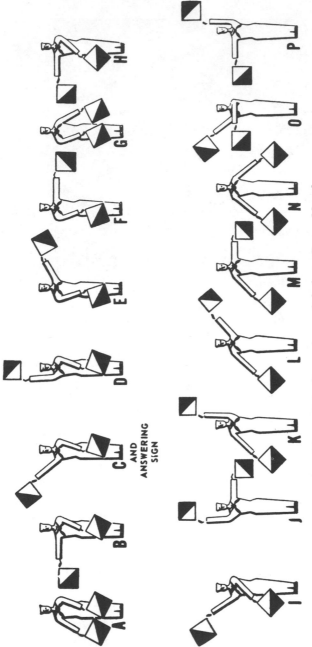

Figure 5-4 Semaphore alphabet. (From *Naval Orientation*, Bureau of Naval Personnel Training Publications Division.)

166

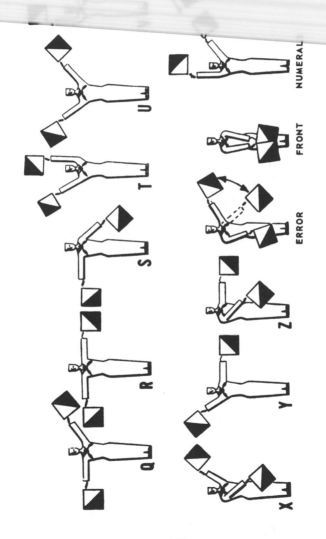

Q R S T U

X Y Z ERROR FRONT NUMERAL

gested fan movements are fanning yourself by shaking it, moving fan from side to side and up and down; extending fan forward as though offering it and then placing it at chest; closing and opening it using two hands and then trying to open and close fan with one hand; bringing arms together and opening and closing arms like a fan; keeping one hand uplifted with the elbow bent and placing opposite hand on elbow, then changing hands; bringing fan close to face and peeking over it.

When many members of the group complain of arthritis or stiffness of the hands, it is sometimes effective to do rhythmic and dramatic activities with hand or finger puppets. These can be faces drawn on old gloves or mittens (even inexpensive "night cream" gloves will do) (Figure 5–5). The actions of opening or closing the hand and using the opposing thumb will create a "mouth" of a dog or other animal. "How Much Is That Doggie In The Window?", "Bingo," or "Old MacDonald Had a Farm" are songs that have added to the fun of hand movements. It is also enjoyable to encourage group members to make finger or hand puppets that can be given to grandchildren or used for dramatic plays among residents or visitors. Puppets can be inexpensively constructed by cutting and folding stiff paper

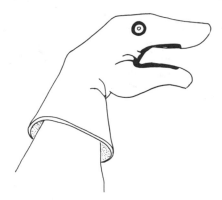

Figure 5-5 Glove hand puppets. Kassoy

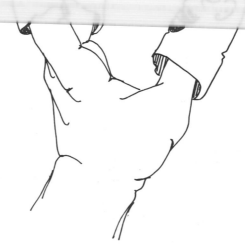

Figure 5-6 Cone finger puppets. Kassoy

into small cones. (The paper cones are made so that they fit snugly on the ends of one's fingers.) Each cone is topped by "heads" made of cotton balls or bits of nylon stockings stuffed with cotton and decorated with faces and hair. These puppets often inspire an increased use of fingers, hands, and arms for the elderly and may also produce some interesting dramatic expression (Figure 5–6).

Rods, wands, cardboard tubes, and other medium-sized sticks can be used to extend movement or to produce accompanying sounds. Many bending and stretching exercises become more challenging if one holds a rod (light-weight, about 14 inches long) in one or both hands and tries to keep the elbows extended or tries to touch various body parts. Elastic "stretch ropes" are familiar accessories for exercise programs and add dimension and resistance to action. *Bath and face towels* are readily available "props" for exercise. They can be used at wash-up time to provide diagonal stretching behind the back and twisting action at the hips and behind the shoulders. Small towels can also be used during group sessions for increasing reaching and bending activities when a towel is held lengthwise with an end in each hand. Wringing and pulling motions with the towel will also assist wrist and shoulder mobility and stimulate static contraction.

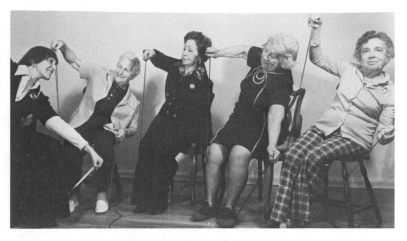

Photo 17   Elastic Stretch Ropes
Robert Blucher

Tapping a *cardboard tube* from a roll of paper toweling on the floor, the chair, a shoulder, and one's hand can be a good way to improve coordination, concentration, and rhythmic response. Group members may suggest some unique ways of responding to march music like "Seventy-six Trombones" or "Alexander's Ragtime Band." Also many classical and modern music selections offer motivation that is appropriate for action with props like these. Slow, strong, stirring, mysterious, or even lyrical accompaniment may be used.

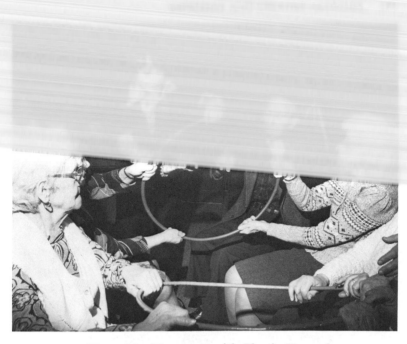

Photo 18 Movement with Plastic Hoops
Mike M. Miyata

We have found that *small plastic hoops* are wonderful aids to movement. For blind or timid clients it is helpful to offer a hoop for two people to share. Hoops are ideal for this purpose if they are approximately 15 inches in diameter and made of lightweight plastic. Many toy or sporting goods stores stock them. They may be made by purchasing narrow gauge plastic garden hose and cutting it to desired lengths and then inserting a 3-inch wooden dowel to connect the two cut ends and then fastening them with heavyweight staples through the hose and the dowel. Ask one person of each duo to be the "leader" and move the hoop in such a fashion that the partner will be able to follow and enjoy the "journey." While holding the hoop, there are opportunities to relax and follow and perhaps experience new movement possibilities and feelings with someone else. Each person should have the chance to initiate the motion as the "leader." Many rewarding sessions have developed with depressed and regressed patients using this technique. And most active groups of older adults also love to take a "hoop trip." It can be done sitting, standing, or moving about the room depending on the participants' capabilities.

Other props that have proved beneficial are light-weight *plastic balls* with attached ribbons or strings that can be used to extend or outline movement of arms and torso. *Plastic Frisbees* or sturdy paper plates (with a 4-inch oblong section cut out near the edge to provide a hand grip) can be held in one or both hands to give more interest and incentive to arm movements. Also, *small flashlights* in a semi-darkened room have stimulated groups to attempt new and increased activity to produce "designs" on the ceiling or walls. We also recommend *sponges* and "nerf" balls (soft sponge balls) to squeeze in the hands, elbow joints, and even knee and hip joints. Men will be especially pleased to use lightweight *rubber balls* (approximately 6 inches in di-ameter) that can be bounced in time with the music or used for throwing and catching alone or with partners. *Homemade weights* such as socks filled with sand, rice, or sugar are useful for lifting activities. Tennis ball cans that are filled with seeds or pebbles can be lifted up and down and side-ward like "dumbbells."

The torsos of some aged individuals are often "fro-zen" like a solid block from long-term inactivity or the tension of pain. Twisting, turning, and rocking may be easier for these people if they sit on an *invalid ring* partially filled with water or air to increase pelvic mobility.

Sometimes there are groups in which individuals are sensually deprived and it is desirable to provide additional stimulation. A chance to touch and use *objects of different textures and physical properties* may be appreciated. We have achieved great success by assembling a "feelie" bag. We offer it as a springboard for movement or discussion ideas. The contents of our "feelie" bag or touch and tell

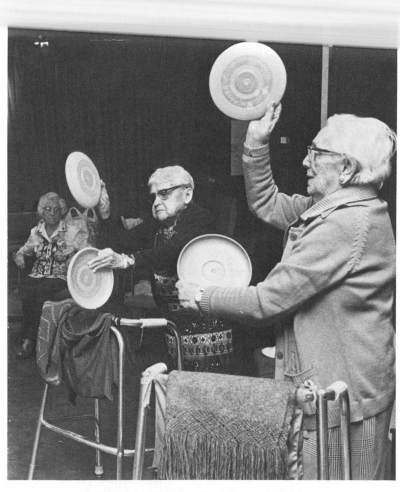

Photo 19   Rhythm Activity with Frisbees
Sam Siegel—Metropolitan Photo Service

collection includes pieces of velvet, satin, and nubby tweed fabric, a large conch shell, a rough rock and a smooth stone, an ostrich feather, a stiff brush, and a piece of "Silly Putty." The sense of smell can also be used to stimulate emotional and movement response by awakening memory traces. Scraps of fabric containing the odors of perfume, garlic, soap, mouthwash, and spices can be used. Additions and deletions are made in response to the group's needs and we are always pleased with the reactions to the varied qualities represented.

Rhythm instruments can also be used to inspire movement and reveal thoughts and emotions that have been pent up. Instead of using them to make music, rattles, drums, and gongs become vehicles through which to express feelings, communicate with someone else, and to manipulate the environment in an acceptable way. We have offered a drum and beater to a nervous, perseverating individual whose extremely limited, repetitive behavior was habitual. After a few sessions the client achieved a unique, strong series of beats with recognizable phrasing. Eventually (12 small-group contacts) the client produced a rhythm with one simple variation that was played with delight. Another patient found great joy in producing long, reverberating sounds on the gong. Many tense older persons are able to externalize their emotions by shaking rattles in angry, fearful, threatening, or even exuberantly joyful ways. A particularly rewarding use of instruments for communication involves bongo drums with depressed or withdrawn clients. We have had "conversations" between therapist and client when the two sit opposite one another and share the drum heads. They respond to the rhythms produced by each other. Sometimes the way to start is to help the patient produce sound by placing his/her hand on the drum nearest and "replying" on your drum and continuing until there is spontaneous action. In order to encourage response, it may be helpful to use the fingertips, fingernails, fists, or

individual longing to release energy, its attention on beating the drum.

Safe and acceptable ways of acting out feelings and concerns may involve using *punch balls* or *bop jollies*, or "Thumper" bats. Even negative feelings will be shared in the safety of a trusting, supportive setting. It is helpful to provide specific limits of boundaries with regard to limits in space so that an individual can express violent

rage, fury, and desperation in rhythmic physical action with inanimate objects. Many limp or tense clients, in addition to seemingly placid ones, have achieved therapeutic release and insight through this activity. Some suggestions we have found effective to contain response include, "Try making contact with the wall in as many ways as you can with the padded thumper bat, keeping time with the music"; "Use the punching bag to show the strong, loud feelings of the music"; "Within a small area, throw the pillow as hard and as high as possible, over and over again"; "Punch the ball as you say angry words, faster and faster."

Images For Self-Expression

Often there are groups or situations in which music is neither possible nor appropriate for the movement session. For these times, the leader-therapist may want to initiate movement by introducing props, such as those objects previously mentioned, or by suggesting vocal or verbal sounds. It may prove fascinating to experiment with rhythms produced by group members such as clicking, humming, grunting, hissing, slapping, snapping, stamping, and so forth. These can all provoke movement responses. In addition, words, poems, and stories may elicit physical action. We've used onamatopoeic words like "crash," "snap, crackle, and pop," "swish," "ping," and descriptive words such as enormous, delicate, and gooey to encourage personal insights and increased movement range. "Motion" words such as flip, sparkle, ooze, whip, slash, and stroke may be said at different intervals as one moves correspondingly. During creative activity, group members can be encouraged to express anger, hostility, joy, or serenity with sounds and words. It may be suitable to say "Bang," "Pow," "Ouch," "Go Away," "Hmmmm," "Ow," "Ooooh," or "Hello." This can create a unity of expression involving the voice and the body to communicate. Poems such as "The Cat" by Carl Sandburg and "Boots" by Rudyard Kipling may also provide sight and sound imagery for self-expression.

Many sense memory and situational studies that are used in drama and pantomime classes may be applied to the therapeutic movement group to stimulate individual response. Those that involve diversity of energy, space, and rhythm include: a scarecrow in a windy field, a snowman under a warm sun, a lion on the prowl, a rattlesnake ready to attack, a contented cat purring, and people that are walking in mud, snow, or water, or stretching out on a sunny beach, pushing a huge boulder, being pushed by a strong wind, banging on a locked door, wandering in an immense space, or being enclosed in a small space. These may be presented with the suggestion that each person try to let his/her muscles put him/her in the picture or situation described. Then one can extend the movements and enlarge on the feelings and ideas that emerge. Sometimes just allowing one part of the body to lead a movement (head, elbow, shoulder, hip, knee) and then trying to let the motion flow from one dominant body part to another will produce a satisfying sequence. The movement can be done slowly and smoothly or quickly and sharply to experience the differences in meaning and sensation.

In order to increase upper torso and arm mobility and to improve overt rhythmic response, the gestures of a musical conductor can be helpful. We start by following the imagery and spatial design of the simplest two beat rhythm with one hand to music. This is usually march or merengue music, and then we progress to three-beat (3/4) waltz or mazurka, and then to four-beat (4/4) marches or jazz tunes. If the group is particularly alert or well coordinated the six-beat (6/8) pattern may be tried (Figure 5-7).

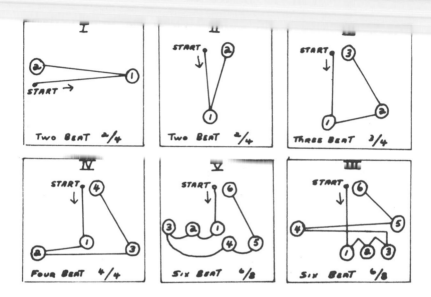

Figure 5-7   "Musical conductors"—spatial designs for
arm movements. A. Rosenthal

Ideas that include oppositional movement factors can produce rewarding individual, dual, and group improvisations. If the leader presents ideas such as "toward and away," "near and far," "high and low," "large and small," "strong and weak," and "slow and fast," the client can easily respond in action. These movements can then be repeated and varied so that increased physical and emotional involvement will result. Mimetic oppositional actions such as pushing and pulling or waving "hello" and "goodbye" can initiate richly expressive dance patterns. Also opening and closing concepts may be transformed from specific gestures (close doors, open windows) to valuable communication.

Two areas of achievement that movement therapists strive for are improved concentration and the establishment of trust. We use dyads for "trust" walks that require each member of the pair to be sensitive and cooperative with each other so that the roles of leading and being led will produce a satisfying experience. One person helps another explore an area (room, corridor) through all the senses except sight. The leader of the pair sees, but the partner closes his/her eyes and accepts the guidance offered. Depending on the physical abilities of the participants, trust walks can be conducted in wheelchairs, walkers, sitting on the floor, or in bed. The opportunity for giving and taking in a couple relationship adds to the benefits of improved sensory awareness and confidence.

Many groups enjoy activity with an imaginary ball. We have mimed ball playing with various-sized balls from golf balls through huge medicine balls. The careful observation and social responsibility involved make this a worthy activity. In a line or a circle, the people can throw, catch, roll, bounce, kick, and dodge an invisible ball that everyone "sees" by imagining and concentrating.

Other springboards for self-expression do not involve objects or word concepts. "Hand dancing" is an opportunity to relate one to one and experience the roles of leader and follower while trying interesting movement patterns. Two people (standing or sitting) face each other and place the palms of their hands together. Designate one person of each pair to be the first leader who will guide the other by the movement of his/her hands to stretch, bend, twist, sway, and so on. The action can be in place or moving around the room and may involve changes of level and direction. It is helpful to keep motion moderately slow and

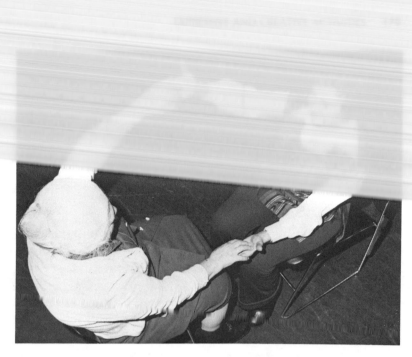

Photo 20   A Trust Experience
Mike M. Miyata

smooth so that it can be followed easily. The contact and concentration between the two participants is a wonderful experience, especially for the aged who know isolation so well.

A variation of hand dancing is the mirror image for passive and active participation. In a one-to-one relationship or with one leader for a small group, one person moves as the initiator and the others reflect as accurately as possible the movement they see. With eye contact only, no verbal communication, there is almost a "magic power" or accepted control at work so that there is an opportunity for the leader to see his/her physical image reflected and actualized and for the follower to experience new movement possibilities and participate in a passive role. There should be opportunities for each participant to try both leading and following and also have a chance to talk about their reactions to the different feelings and situations. Slow, sustained music may prove appropriate to most groups. However, we have also found that moderately bouncy or staccato selections may encourage some groups, who might be reluctant, to try the activity as a marionette and string puller for an initial experience.

Musical Instruments and Rhythm Games

IMPORTANCE OF RHYTHM INSTRUMENTS.   The movement therapist may be fortunate to work in a facility that has an extensive staff of creative therapists, including music specialists, and so provides programming and equipment for a rich therapeutic experience. But many circumstances are not ideal and there is a need for activities and therapeutic personnel to work cooperatively and creatively to provide as diverse a program as possible. Group singing and music listening opportunities are often led by volunteers and the leader of geriatric dance/movement sessions may find it necessary to provide the means for producing music through rhythmic activity. Simple percussion instruments like those found in children's rhythm bands are ideal for older people. They provide a reasonable challenge physically and mentally, they produce clear rhythmic beats, and they stimulate group response and interaction. The production of shared sounds is very enjoyable to elderly groups.

It is essential that the instruments be presented as music makers and not toys. The beneficial results derived from their use should be emphasized.

TYPES OF APPROPRIATE RHYTHM INSTRUMENTS.   For economy and practicality, percussion instruments can be made from easily available objects. Plastic buckets can be drums; macaroni or seeds in small containers become rattles; and spoons or sticks can be rhythm sticks. An ideally diverse collection of instruments should include cymbals (large and small finger types), triangles, maracas, castanets, tambourines, gongs, bells, whistles, drums, and xylophones or autoharps. But a limited selection can still be adequate when used by an inventive leader. (See pages 293 and 294 on selection and purchase of instruments.)

When older persons have difficulty grasping or holding an object for long periods of time, it may be helpful to provide elastic bracelets or bands to slip over the hands rather than the ordinary grip handles provided on cymbals or bells.

PLAYING RHYTHM INSTRUMENTS.

1. The leader-therapist selects a musical recording and the group plays instruments in response to the strongly accented beats. "Masquerade," a traditional folk dance

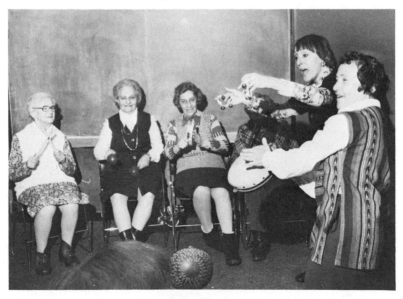

Photo 21   Playing Rhythm Instruments
Mike M. Miyata

tune (MH 1019B Folkdancer Records), has three distinctly different sections in which the music has 4/4, then 3/4, and finally 2/4 time. These sections are repeated at regular four-measure intervals throughout the recording and provide varied qualities for the elderly group to accompany. The members can be divided into three sections. Each section is given a different type of instrument to play and then they wait for one particular four-measure musical phrase to accompany:

4/4- use drums or rhythm sticks

3/4- use triangles or bells

2/4- use maraccas (rattles)

2.   Often, it is an enjoyable challenge for groups to respond vocally or with claps or stamps to the signal of a musical phrase. Songs like "Deep in the Heart of Texas," "Finjan," "Mexican Waltz," and "La Raspa" lend themselves to this kind of participation.

3.   "Conversational" playing provides a good opportunity for self-expression. Instruments are used to "speak" to someone else. One person plays and another person listens and then responds. This can be accomplished by sharing the same instrument (photo 22), or by using individual instruments. There can be questions and answers, friendly counterpoint, or an angry conflict with the sounds of instrument "voices."

4.   A variation of having a conversation with percussion instruments is to use the instrument to portray a type of person or an emotion. For instance, try to produce sounds that are happy, lighthearted, stern, foolish, frightened, calm, and so on.

5.   A good socializing activity with instruments is to use half of the pair of cymbals per person and then play them together. This involves concentration and cooperation and can be done with duos of group members or between the leader and a client.

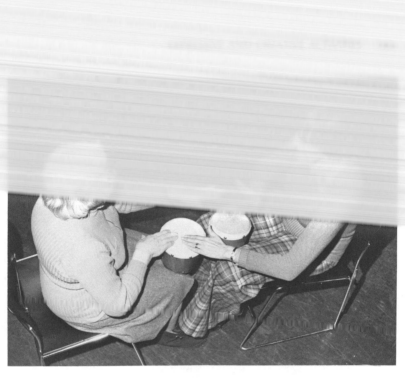

Photo 22 Conversation with Bongo Drums
Mike M. Miyata

6. Echoing is another technique of working with instruments. The therapist or leader plays a rhythm and the
group repeats or echoes what it hears. This can be made
more challenging and interesting, after the group has mas-
tered the concentration involved, by asking for echoes that
are softer or louder than the original or slower or faster
than the leader has played. (The original rhythmic pattern
must be maintained with regard to accents and relationships of note values.)

Metrical accompaniment (example on page 181) is the
most common way of playing rhythm instruments in time
with a musical recording. The leader-therapist chooses music that is appropriate to the group and that also provides
a strongly accented beat that can be followed easily. Tan-
gos, marches, folk tunes, and popular melodies such as
"Syncopated Clock" are good selections for rhythmic ac-

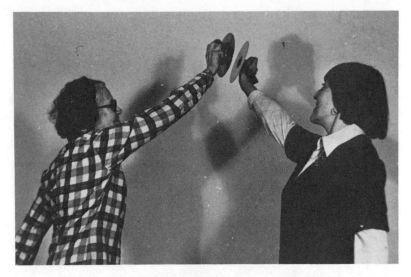

Photo 23   Playing Cymbals for Socialization
Robert Blucher

companiment. It is possible to have unison playing, which is quite satisfying if the music is interesting and pleasing for the group. When additional challenge is desirable, two- or three-party playing may be suggested. This entails dividing the group into sections and each takes a turn playing at a different time.

7.   If the music selected has a chorus-stanza form, then it is possible to have half the people play the stanza (or verse) and the other half play the chorus (refrain).

8.   Another organizational suggestion is to have as many small groups as there are stanzas in the song so that everyone plays for each repeated chorus, but one small group at a time plays for each stanza in turn.

9.   It may also be enjoyable, if the music chosen is slow enough, to have one group play the strong accents and another group play the weaker beats. For example, the rhythm sticks could beat on count 1, and the rattles could play 2 and 3 during a slow waltz.

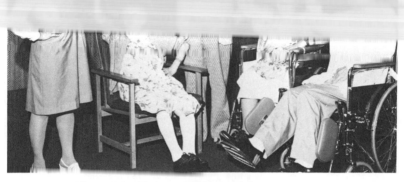

Photo 24   Unison Playing with Instruments
Mike M. Miyata

10.   It is often beneficial for groups to use their instruments in conjunction with exercises so they bend and stretch as they play in time to the music. In this instance the strong beats of the music and the accent of the movement are accompanied by the sound of the rhythm instruments.

RHYTHM GAMES.   The following games are effective with older groups because the important elements are relaxation, enjoyment, and socialization. There is careful avoidance of competitive elements of winning and losing and the skills involved are uncomplicated. Emphasis is placed on concentration, observation, and cooperation within acceptable levels of stimulation. Everyone is encouraged to participate since there are no special skills involved, and people are not "eliminated" or losers, but achieve something at different stages of the game. When objects are passed from one person to another the rhythmic and physical action is important, but equally beneficial is the chance to reinforce one's focusing of attention.

Formations for games can be very important and yet difficult to achieve. This is especially true if the group is not ambulatory or is very heterogeneous. We have found many variations of the standard line and circle necessary. Figure 5–8 shows some that proved effective.

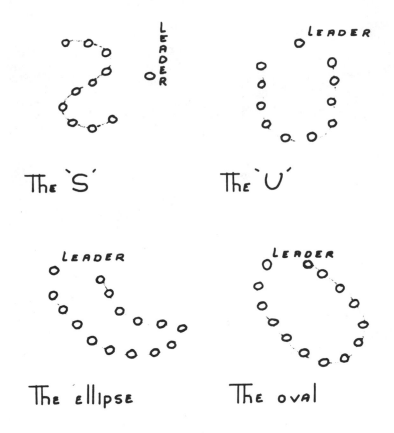

Figure 5-8   Group formations. A. Rosenthal

Individual Activity

1.   The leader has a game ball and gives it to each patient who then bounces it back to the leader. A particularly alert and well-coordinated patient will be able to throw the ball in the air and catch it or pass it from one hand to the other before bouncing it back to the leader.

2.   One large cardboard carton is placed in front of a small group of participants, each of whom has a bean bag. On a designated signal from the leader, one person at a time throws the bean bag into the box with a strong, propulsive movement of arm and hand. Heavily accented musical accompaniment such as "The Anvil Chorus," "Volga Boatman," "Hall of the Mountain King," or "Praise the Lord and Pass the Ammunition" are appropriate. The leader may also play a drum with a rhythmic phrase that has rapid, soft beats and at the end of the phrase play one loud, strong beat that is the signal for the throwing of the bean bag. Repeat the rhythmic phrase until each person has thrown the bean bag into the box. Then the leader picks up the box, gives the bean bags back, and moves the box further away from the group.

Group Activity   We have discovered that the following version of the classic, "Musical Chairs," may be a delightful way to distribute scarves or rhythm sticks in addition to providing rhythmic play.

1.   Group members are seated close to each other, preferably in a circle. A rhythm stick or a scarf is passed from person to person as the music plays. When the leader stops the music, the person holding the object keeps it and places it in his/her lap. When the music resumes, a new stick or scarf is passed. Continue stopping and starting until everyone has an object. A person does not keep more than one object. This is appropriate for alert, well, elderly groups.

2.   One tambourine or bean bag is passed in a clockwise direction from person to person while the music plays. When the leader signals, with a clap or a spoken direction, whoever is holding the object starts passing it in the opposite direction. A song like "Pop Goes The Weasel" can be used and on "pop" change direction.

3.   With a large, light beach ball the level of the passing can be changed at the signal. For example, start passing the ball from one to another person at chest height, then when the leader claps change to passing below the knees.

4.   With a particularly alert group, it is possible to alter the method of passing from person to person in a follow the leader fashion each time the signal is given. Suggestions include receiving with one hand and changing it to the other hand and then passing to the next person; receiving with one hand and passing across the body to the next person; passing the object behind back; adding hand clapping or foot stamping while passing; or ball bouncing before passing. Music that has worked well for this activity includes "Syncopated Clock," "Alexander's Ragtime Band," "Turkey in the Straw," and "Seventy-six Trombones."

5.   A ball or bean bag is passed around the group in time to the music. At a signal, the person holding the ball throws it into a large box that the leader holds or that is placed in front of the group member. Then the ball is retrieved and the music and the passing resumes.

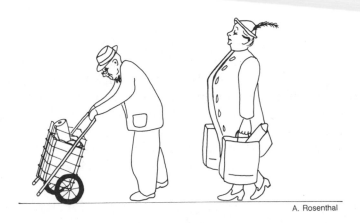

A. Rosenthal

GUIDANCE BY THE LEADER-THERAPIST

The role of the leader-therapist, which includes more than directing movement activities, involves elements of guidance and counseling. There are opportunities to help the participant form a positive outlook through techniques of acceptance and clarification. Group discussion in a permissive and encouraging atmosphere helps older adults to see that their problems are not unique. They are comforted by sharing common concerns.

Sometimes topics are brought up by a client's questions. Others are introduced by the leader because of observation during that particular session. They may also be gathered from cues presented over an extended period of time.

In some groups there may even be individuals with valuable professional and practical experience that can be shared and appreciated by their peers. At the Jewish Home and Hospital for the Aged in New York City, a few blind patients were brought in to join the regular movement therapy group. During the activity, one of the newcomers kept constantly protesting in a negative manner, saying, "What am I doing here? Take me out. . . ." When one of the aides approached her she said angrily, "Don't touch me!" The leader ignored her for a time and continued with the session, which was now concerned with offering helpful hints on the activities of daily living. Suddenly her voice was heard giving suggestions also. The therapist paid close attention to what she said and encouraged her to continue. The whole group listened attentively to her advice and discovered that she had been an orthopedic nurse. She thus became interested in group concerns and said she would be happy to return the following week and join the group.

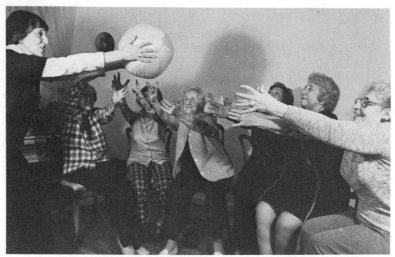

Photo 25   Rhythm Game with Ball
Robert Blucher

that they evolve in a more or less spontaneous way. Discussion may be stimulated at the start, as the session progresses, or it can be saved for the conclusion, whenever it is most appropriate.

GENERAL HEALTH AND SAFETY ISSUES

Significance of Body Alignment

The spine provides the support for all the vital organs. Sometimes people feel comfortable in sitting or standing positions that are really harmful to them. The body makes adjustments to maintain balance and continue functioning, which may require more work or cause unhealthy conditions.

If the head and neck are not in line with the other parts of the body, if they are thrust forward or off-balance, then swallowing, coughing, and even speech will be more difficult.

The upper spine, between the shoulders and the waist, supports the heart, lungs, and diaphragm. Slumping or slouching restricts breathing and makes it harder for the heart to work well. Even for people who are restricted to chairs, the lift of the head and the chest literally improves their outlook on the world.

The position of the lower back and hips affects the circulation and the support of the organs that control good digestion and regular elimination.

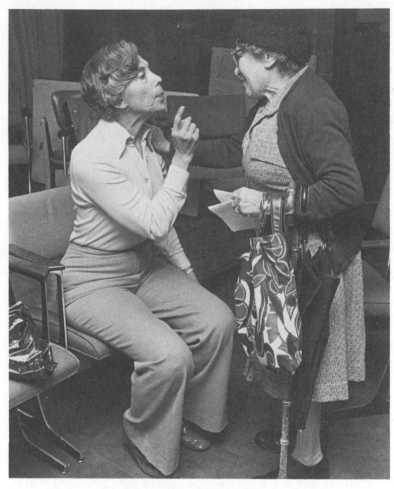

Photo 26   Giving Advice
Sam Siegel—Metropolitan Photo Service

The spinal column encloses the spinal chord, which is a control center for many of the nerves of the body. Thus pain and lowered energy can result from pressure caused by a shortened or twisted spine.

The legs and feet are also important to good body position and function because the feet are the foundations for the body, muscles according to status. They must be firmly in contact with the chair and in a direct line with the knees to provide good balance.

In order to feel good about oneself and maintain healthy functioning, one should be aware of the importance of keeping the various parts of the body in proper relationships to each other (Figure 6-1).

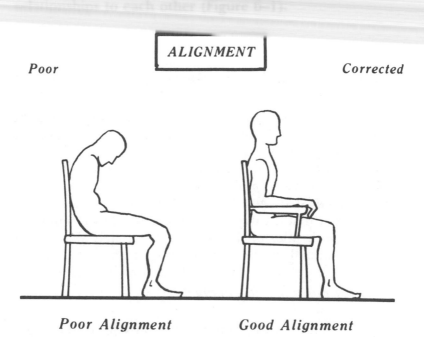

Figure 6-1   Good and poor alignment. (From *Elementary Rehabilitation Nursing Care,* U. S. Public Health Service, Division of Nursing.)

Sitting Considerations

The life of the elderly person is often sedentary (card playing, television viewing, etc.) and therefore the construction of the chairs used is important for safety, comfort, and health. The chairs that are appropriate for the older adult are sturdy with a firm seat that is the right height and depth so that the person's feet can be placed firmly on the floor and his/her lower spine can be against the chair back (Figure 6–2).

It is better for circulation and for muscle tone if one sits in a firm, straightbacked chair without crossing the legs at the knees.

To minimize deterioration due to inactivity, hours spent sitting should be interspersed with intervals of stretching, standing, and/or walking around.

Carrying and Lifting Precautions

Always turn to face the surface on which an object is to be placed or lifted from, in order to avoid injury from twisting or falling off balance.

Hold objects in the arms close to the body, rather than carrying a heavy shopping bag dragging from one hand. This reduces stress for the shoulder, neck, and arm joints.

Weight that is carried can be balanced by holding objects on both sides of the body or alternately shifting the weight from side to side, minimizing strain.

Hints for Pushing and Pulling

It is more efficient to use the strong muscles of the thighs rather than the back or shoulder muscles when exerting force. Therefore, one must bend at the knees and at the hips while grasping with the hands for such activities as pushing and pulling. The body should lean in the direction of the energy and movement desired.

Importance of Securing Assistance

Older people are often isolated and impatient and so they overtax themselves by attempting tasks that are too diffi-

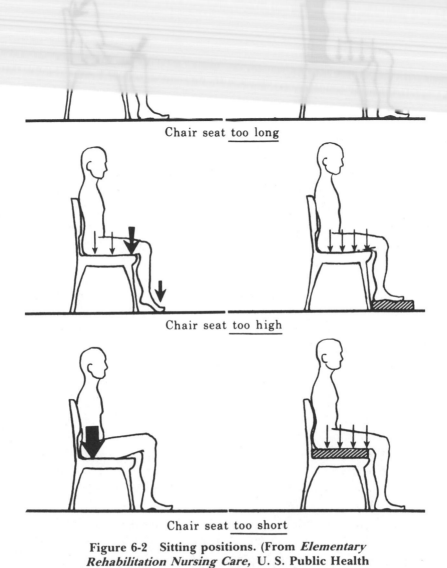

Chair seat too long

Chair seat too high

Chair seat too short

Figure 6-2   Sitting positions. (From *Elementary Rehabilitation Nursing Care,* U. S. Public Health Service, Division of Nursing.)

cult. It is essential to encourage senior citizens to use one of the prerogatives of age and ask for assistance in order to:

Move heavy objects such as furniture.

Carry bulky items like big marketing orders.

Reach high places such as the top of curtain rods and closet shelves.

Precautions for Bathing

All bathing facilities for the aged should provide handrails and nonslip surfaces for stability. Showering is less precarious for the elderly, especially if a sturdy, skidproof stool is provided so that one can sit to avoid fatigue. The use of nonskid floor mats (never towels) is an important precaution for everyone, particularly the elderly. Also maintaining a moderate water temperature is a safety factor to avoid fainting, dizziness, or decreased visibility that might be caused by steam or extremes of heat or cold.

Older citizens who are independent and active enough to bathe themselves need to establish a careful routine of movements that will make it possible to execute the complicated maneuvers of entering and leaving a bathtub safely. (See pages 211, 212.)

Special Aids and Activities for Arthritis, Stroke, Parkinson's Disease, Incontinence, and Digestive Difficulties

Regular participation in activities to maintain or increase the range of motion should be encouraged for all elderly persons. Extensive evidence is now available to indicate the physiological, psychological, and social benefits of physical exercise for both well and disabled older adults. Dr. Brice

thusiastic acceptance of physical activity programs by the members of the medical profession" (33). Many of our group members remark that the movements that we encourage are similar to those recommended by their physicians.

There are special exercises to aid in the normal body functions such as elimination, respiration, circulation, and muscular tone. And with improved functioning, many of the common disabling conditions of old age can be alleviated.

ARTHRITIS.   Most elderly individuals have periodic attacks of rheumatoid or osteoarthritis, but some suffer from progressive pain and joint changes. During acute periods of joint inflammation the doctor may order temporary rest. Then relaxation and breathing sequences should be the only activities indulged in until the acute stage passes. Positioning the joints in mild extension, warm water soaks, moist heat compresses, passive exercises (no more than five repeats for each), plus massage are often helpful for the arthritic patient.

The following exercises are suggested for improving the flexibility of troublesome joints.

In a back-lying position:

1.   With arms around one leg, bring that knee up toward the chest, then bring it back to starting position.

Repeat with the other leg and then bring both knees toward chest with the arms around them and then relax.

2.   Bring both knees toward chest with arms clasped around them and gently rock back and forth on back.

In a kneeling position with hands on floor (on all fours):

3.   Like a cat stretching, round the back with the head down and pull the abdominal muscles in as the hips tuck under. Then arch the back, lifting the head upward. Maintain extended elbows throughout the activity (Figures 6–3 and 6–4).

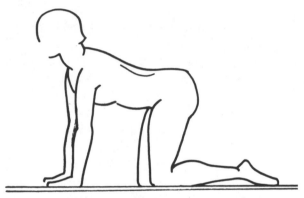

Figure 6-3   Kneeling position on all fours. Kassoy

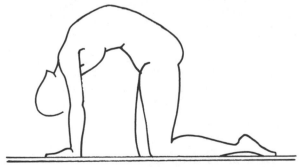

Figure 6-4   Cat stretch. Kassoy

4. Place one hand against a wall and slowly attempt to extend the arm upward as though climbing. (Fingers may slide or "creep" up the wall.)

5. Press hands together with palms touching and try to bend the fingers of one hand backward with the heel of the opposing hand. Alternate hands (Figure 6–5).

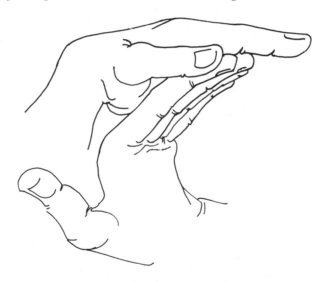

Figure 6-5   Hand press. Kassoy

6. With one hand at a time and then attempt with both: touch tip of thumb with the tip of the first, then second, then third, and then little finger in turn (Figure 6–6).

Moving thumb out and around to touch little finger.

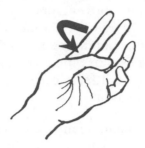

Opposition

Figure 6-6   Thumb in opposition. (From *Elementary Rehabilitation Nursing Care*, U. S. Public Health Service, Division of Nursing.)

7.   Circle the hands by rotating at the wrists, then with hand extended palm upward, bend wrist so palm faces forearm, then return hand to starting position (Figure 6–7).

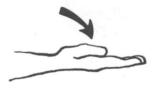   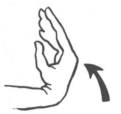

Extension   Flexion

Figure 6-7   Flexion and extension. (From *Elementary Rehabilitation Nursing Care*, U. S. Public Health Service, Division of Nursing.)

8.   Hold a sponge or a ball in one or both hands and squeeze slowly and as strongly as possible and then relax hands.

9.   Clasp hands together with interlocked fingers, palms down. Then lift elbows and wrists to produce an extension of the finger joints. Then stretch the arms for-

sions, and some "homework" practices, she reported enthusiastically to the group without her bandage (just warm cotton stockings), "I got up on the bus yesterday by myself; getting down—that's a different story!"

When the elbows and fingers are very painful, it may be helpful to carefully heat bean bags in the oven or on a radiator and then place them at the elbows or hold them in the hands as one bends or extends the joints. (Moist warm compresses are even more beneficial, but are usually less convenient during exercise. Activity in a warm pool or bath, with supervision, may be ideal.)

To overcome excessive flexion and cramping of fingers and hands, which precludes holding objects, some adaptations can be made. We have discovered that musical instruments are used successfully by arthritic patients when loose elastic bands are attached to cymbals, or bells are sewn onto circles of wide elastic webbing. Then the instruments can be "worn" around the center of the hand. The patient is able to join in the rhythmic activity without the need to grip something for any length of time.

STROKE.   Neuromuscular impairment resulting from cardiovascular accidents is prevalent among the aged population. It is desirable to maintain mobility in the unaffected limbs and so activities with the strong as well as the weak areas of the body should be included when working with the poststroke individual. The stroke patient can be encouraged to participate with his/her unaffected body parts and also to use the strong limbs, when possible, to assist the weaker ones. Movements may be done in lying or sitting positions.

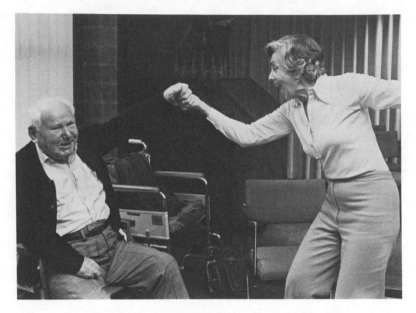

Photo 27   Encouraging the Stroke Patient
Sam Siegel—Metropolitan Photo Service

Because of problems of balance and control, the stroke patient is often limited to activity of the limbs alone. Therefore the leader-therapist must offer movement variety to avoid repetition and fatigue. This can be done through changes of energy and range of motion. For example, in addition to raising and lowering the arms or legs one can flex and extend, shake, circle, swing, and rotate.

Some passive range-of-motion exercises that have proved to be helpful are:

1. Use the strong hand to lift the affected arm in different directions.

The same procedure may be applied to the legs in sitting or lying positions. Place the foot of the strong leg behind the ankle of the weak one, and lift the weak leg as high as possible and lower it gently (Figure 6-8).

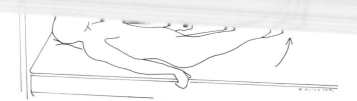

Figure 6-8   Use of strong limb to lift weaker one. A. Rosenthal

3.   Place the healthy hand on the elbow of the affected arm and gently pull the elbow toward the center of the body to encourage shoulder mobility, then release.

4.   Shrugging or lifting and lowering of the shoulders may help to relax spasticity through released tension.

5.   With elbows bent and hands interlocked in front of chest, rotate torso and move arms sideward (Figure 6–9).

PARKINSON'S DISEASE.   This disability, characterized by tremors, rigidity, and loss of motor function, ranks third after cerebral vascular disease and arthritis as the most common chronic disease of the aged (34).

1.   Dance patterns to such songs as "Hokey Pokey" (see page 145) and "Alley Cat" (EA32, Educational Activities Record) are good to improve static and dynamic balance.

2.   Rhythmic hand clapping and instrument playing aid in maintaining coordination and reciprocity patterns (see pages 181–185).

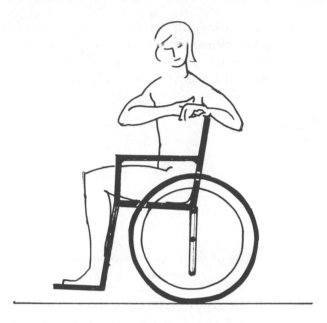

Figure 6-9   Rotating torso with interlocked hands.
Kassoy

3. Games like Hot Potato which can be done to the recording of "Syncopated Clock" (AR85; Educational Activities Record) and other passing activities with wands and balls or tossing and catching with bean bags will be beneficial (see pages 185–188).

4. Squeezing paper towels or napkins, range of motion exercises such as those recommended for arthritis (page 000–000), and marching actions will help mobility.

5. To counteract facial rigidity and speech problems, patients can try smiling, frowning, puffing out the cheeks, pointing and curling the tongue, and moving the jaw from side to side. Also see exercises on pages 80, 93, and 100.

INCONTINENCE.   Many elderly people who suffer from a bowel or urinary weakness due to poor muscle tone can benefit from the practice of conscious muscle control.

These exercises may be done in sitting, standing, or lying positions. If using the lying position, should be on the back with the knees bent and the feet placed on the reclining surface (see Figure 4-21). Incontinence due to neurological disorders or other impairments will rarely respond to the following muscular conditioning.

1.   Tense the buttocks muscles and maintain this position for five counts. Relax and then repeat.

2.   After tensing buttocks muscles, concentrate on pulling in and lifting up the sphincter muscles of the anus.

3.   In a back-lying position, raise the hips off the bed by contracting the buttocks muscles.

4.   Tighten the muscles in the pelvic area and squeeze the thighs together while concentrating on pulling in and lifting up the urinary sphincter muscles.

Some female clients can practice urinary control by consciously stopping and starting the flow of urine when they are toileting. This will help identify the muscle action desired and provide reinforcement for conscious control.

DIGESTIVE DIFFICULTIES.   Often elderly people are troubled by indigestion, excessive gas, and constipation, which may be due to poor muscle tone and improper diet. Restrictions caused by limited finances, loneliness, and misconceptions prevent the aged from enjoying balanced meals. It is essential to provide the environment and the resources so that a variety of nourishing food is available each day. Smaller amounts of food may be eaten as one ages if the calorie needs decrease because of lowered activity. Nonetheless, each of the four important food groups should be represented in every meal: skim milk and milk products, fruits and vegetables, bread and whole grain cereals, and protein from beans, eggs, fish, poultry, or meat. Good eating patterns must be stressed to help maintain and even restore one's health.

If one is sedentary, the muscles of the abdomen, diaphragm, buttocks, and legs become weak and the circulatory and respiratory systems receive little stimulation and so they are not able to help with digestive functioning.

Exercises such as the following will help individuals get relief from flatulence and improve digestion.

In a sitting position:

1.   With two hands around one knee, lift knee slowly toward chest and then lower leg. Repeat with other leg.
2.   Fold arms across abdomen and press in while bending forward from the hips. Return to erect sitting position.

In a back-lying position:

3.   Bend knees and place feet on floor, then raise hips toward ceiling (like a bridge) by using buttocks and thigh muscles. Then slowly lower hips and draw in stomach muscles as spine returns to the floor (Figure 6–10).

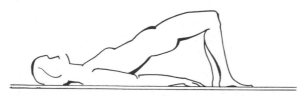

Figure 6-10   Creating a bridge. Kassoy

TECHNIQUES FOR ACTIVITIES OF DAILY LIVING

Because of the high number of accidents sustained by older persons, there is special need for caution and specific suggestions of safe ways to perform daily activities.

Getting into a Chair.

To provide additional support or security, a chair can be positioned in front of the person, with that chair's back facing the chair to be sat upon. The hands can be placed on the chair back.

1.   Place the feet slightly apart with one foot in front of the other, so that the back foot is close to the chair.
2.   Extend the hands to the arms or seat of the chair to provide support.
3.   Then, with spine erect, bend the knees and lower the hips to the seat (Figure 6–11).
4.   Ease back until the lower spine is against the chair back (Figure 6–11).

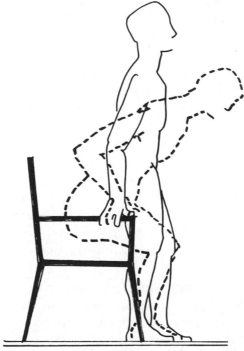

Figure 6-11   Getting into a chair. Kassoy

Getting Out of a Chair

1. Place one foot behind the other under the chair seat.
2. Press hands against chair seat or arms.
3. Bring body forward to the edge of chair seat.
4. Lean forward slightly, without rounding back, so that body weight is over feet.
5. Rise up out of the chair while pushing down with hands and feet.

Climbing Steps

Stairclimbing is excellent exercise to provide conditioning for cardiorespiratory function. The individual who is in good health can step onto buses and ascend staircases with efficiency using the following directions:

1. Place one hand on the handrail.
2. Lift one foot and place it on the step ahead.
3. Transfer body weight to that foot while pressing hand on the handrail.
4. Repeat with alternating feet, one step at a time, keeping body in a slightly diagonal line moving forward and upward.

For frail, disabled, or insecure persons, the use of a one-sided, single step climb is recommended. This is a much safer and less-demanding procedure.

1. Hold banister with hand closest to it.
2. Lift one foot and place it on the step ahead.
3. Press down on the banister with hand while bringing the other foot up beside the first.
4. Continue to climb one step at a time.

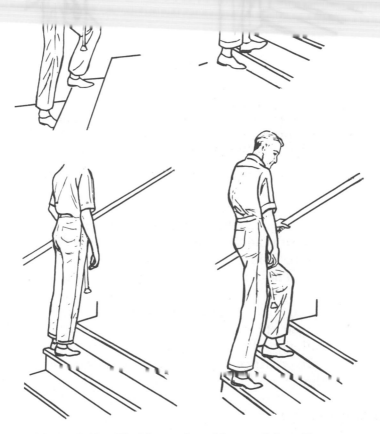

Figure 6-12   Climbing stairs with a weak leg. (From
Up and Around, Heart Disease Control Program,
Division of Chronic Diseases, U. S. Public Health
Service, U. S. Department of Health, Education and
Welfare.)

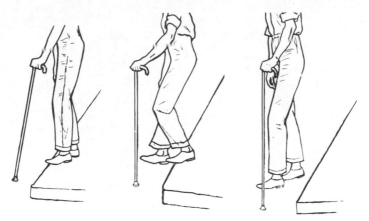

Figure 6-13   Walking down the stairs. (From *Up and Around,* Heart Disease Control Program, Division of Chronic Diseases, U. S. Public Health Service, U. S. Department of Health, Education and Welfare.)

If one leg is injured or weaker than the other:

1. To go up the stairs, lift the strong leg up to the step first and then bring the weak one up next to it. (Use a cane on the side of the stronger leg.) (See Figure 6–12.)
2. Try to hold a handrail on the side of the stronger leg.
3. When walking down stairs, place the weaker leg on the step first, then lower the body weight slowly, as the good leg is placed on the same step. (Use a cane or crutch on the side of the weaker leg.) (See Figure 6–13.)

Lifting an Object

This procedure utilizes the leg muscles rather than putting strain on the more vulnerable back. If the object is heavy for the individual, it should never be lifted above waist height.

Getting Into a Bathtub

1. Turn with side to the tub and grasp the nearest rim of the tub or handrail with the hand on the side furthest away (Figure 6–14).
2. Raise the leg nearest the tub and place the foot securely into the tub while reaching with the hand nearest the tub toward the handle opposite.

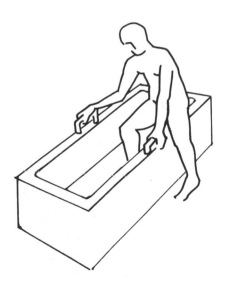

Figure 6-14   Getting into a bathtub. Kassoy

3. Then, with both hands grasping firmly, step into the tub with the other foot.
4. Bend the knees while pressing down on the handles, and lower the body into the tub.

Getting Out of a Bathtub

1. Sitting in the tub, bend both knees up and place them, one on top of the other, to one side.
2. Then turn torso to face outside of tub while placing both hands on same rim or handrail.
3. Press hands downward while rising onto knees.
4. Then step onto one foot and then the other, still maintaining a firm grasp with both hands in front of body.
5. Slowly extend knees to standing and then turn carefully to hold handgrips on both sides of the tub with one hand each.
6. Step out of tub with leg nearest the outside. When foot is securely on the floor, then replace hands so that both are on the outside tub rim.
7. Then raise the other leg to step over the tub side to the floor.

Recommended Sleep Positions

A great proportion of an elderly person's time may be spent in bed. Therefore it is essential to have a firm mattress to support the body so that it can maintain a healthy position and receive a good rest.

If a person has been comfortable and sleeps well in his/her customary position, by all means don't change it. If one finds it difficult to sleep or wakes up with aches and pains, then perhaps he/she would benefit from sleeping in one of the following positions. These do not place any strain on any part of the body and do not interfere with circulation.

side-lying position, sometimes called the climbing position, with one knee bent over the other partially extended leg. To eliminate neck discomfort it might be helpful to place a small cushion under the head and neck (Figures 6–15,16).

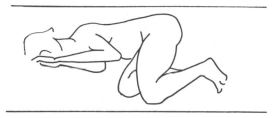

Figure 6-15   Curled sleeping position. Kassoy

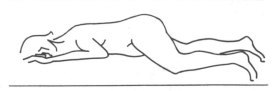

Figure 6-16   Climbing sleeping position. Kassoy

One of our clients related her experience showing the importance of sleeping with good body alignment. Mrs. A. told us: "For the last few years I have awakened with a stiff neck, pain in my shoulders and a backache. I went to several doctors who took X-rays and found nothing wrong with me. Recently, I began to attend your movement sessions at the senior citizens center. Now that I tried your suggestions for sleeping positions, I wake up with almost no pain."

Arising from Sleep

Upon awakening it is important to take time to get out of bed in order to avoid dizziness or loss of balance. Because the body has been relaxed for a number of hours, all of the body functions have slowed down and it is desirable to make a slow, gradual return to activity rather than an abrupt one.

While still lying down, spend a few minutes stretching and yawning. Come up very slowly to a sitting position with the feet dangling over the side of the bed. Slowly place the feet firmly on the floor and then stand up.

Getting Into a Car

Ideally, the car is positioned so that there is space between the car and the curb, so that the elderly person can step down to street level in order to enter the car.

1. Standing at street level, turn the back to the car doorway, place hands on car seat, and then ease body down to the car seat with hips leading, using same procedure as getting into a chair.
2. Hold onto dashboard from front seat or back of front seat if sitting in rear of car, and draw legs into car while shifting hips to face front of car.

Getting Out of a Car

The car is positioned at least two feet away from the curb.

1. Shift the hips to allow the leg nearest to the door to slide out.
2. Continue shifting the body until facing the car doorway to allow other leg to slide out.

We have found that members of therapeutic movement groups ask about specific concerns. These questions can offer opportunities for reassurance, explanation, and referral.

All of the following questions have a medical aspect and so a physician should be consulted if any of these concerns are persistent or severe. Clients should be consistently encouraged to seek medical advice.

"What shall I do if an activity hurts me?"

Stop! Each person is an individual and we all work within our own capabilities.

"I can't do many of the movements because I get tired easily. Should I bother coming to the sessions?"

Yes. Whatever you do, however limited, is better than doing nothing. You only do as much as you can. Not every person participates in everything. Stop when you get tired or join in only for the breathing and relaxation exercises. Enjoy being part of the group.

"How can our movement sessions help painful and stiff joints?"

Movement improves mobility and may retard further deterioration of the joints. Doing the bending, extending, and rotating activities from our sessions when in the bathtub, whirlpool, or after application of warm, moist compresses may be helpful.

"Should I wear a corset when I exercise?"

If you can participate without a corset, that is preferable. Otherwise, wear an old one that is not tight and restricting.

"What can therapeutic movement sessions do for headaches?"

Headaches can be due to many causes. If stress and anxiety are the reasons for the headache, then diversion, relaxation, and an outlet for feelings are provided by the sessions. If the discomfort is due to pressure affecting circulation or nerves, then opportunities to use the muscles of the neck and face, and to change positions of the head may reduce the strain.

"Are there things that I can do to help me fall asleep more easily?"

Usually it is extremely difficult to fall asleep if one is over-stimulated by food or drink. Also when one is anxious or tense, then the mind and body can't relax enough to sleep restfully. Trying the relaxation and breathing techniques from our sessions will be beneficial. Perhaps being more flexible about the selection of bedtime hours will help also.

"What can I do if I wake up at night and can't go back to sleep?"

Many elderly people nap or rest during the day and are not physically or mentally tired enough to sleep through the night. When one wakes up in the middle of the night, instead of lying there and becoming anxious and irritated, it is better to change positions, read, or get out of bed for activity or a warm drink.

"Is there anything you can suggest for constipation?"

Diet that includes fruit and roughage such as salads and whole grains encourages elimination. Activity is impor-

tone the circulation and to stimulate digestion. Specific
exercises for the sphincter muscles of the anus and the
abdominal area will improve the ability to evacuate.

"Shall I exercise with a heart condition?"

Evidence is readily available to show that sedentary, physically inactive living may be a major factor in bringing on
heart disease, and that exercise contributes to the main-

tenance of the psychological, social, and physical well-
being of the individual. And so participation in rhythmic
activities such as relaxation, mild calisthenics, and dancing may be acceptable to your medical advisor. However,
if a graded fitness program to counteract or prevent
heart disease is desired, then a thorough cardiac assessment should be made and special centers for cardiorespiratory training should be utilized (35). Supervised programs have been established at places like Montefiore
Hospital in New York, which offers a postcardiac exercise
regimen. "Y's" and community centers and other hospitals throughout the country provide fitness programs.

"Is exercise alright if one has a pacemaker?"

A regular member of our group has a pacemaker. She has
told us that: "My doctor is pleased to know that I am
keeping in good physical condition because I regularly
join in the sitting exercises and relaxation activities with
the movement and music group."

"How does physical activity affect diabetes?"

Vigorous physical activity may lower the blood sugar level
so that diabetics on insulin should check with their physicians to see if their insulin requirements have decreased.
It is desirable for a diabetic to have a cup of orange juice
or some hard, sucking candies readily available in the
event that one feels weak or faint during exercising.

"Can I do something to help emphysema or an asthmatic problem?"

Yes. The relaxation and breathing techniques mentioned on pages 108 to 116 are often helpful in addition to moderate or passive exercises that stimulate respiratory function.

"What can I do to relieve the discomfort of varicose veins in my legs?"

In order to reduce the pressure of blood in the veins of the legs which causes the discomfort, one should avoid standing still for long periods of time or sitting with the legs crossed at the knee or pressed against the chair seat. Support stockings or elastic bandages may offer some relief and stroking or gentle massage from the ankle toward the heart may be soothing. Activities or resting in a lying position in which the legs are elevated is very beneficial to stimulate the return of blood toward the heart.

"I often get muscle cramps or knots; is there anything I can do?"

Muscle spasms often result in severe pain and limitation of movement. It is important to speak with your physician to determine the cause and possible medical treatment. Symptomatic treatment with a hot pack or warm soaks may decrease the suffering and restore normal motion. Do not attempt activity or weight bearing until the pain is relieved. Then, gentle movements such as massaging, swinging, or slow reaching and bending to return the muscles to normal length and relaxation are helpful.

"I'd like to do massage for myself at home. How would you suggest I try?"

A good time and place for self-massage is when you are bathing. If your bathtub has a nonskid mat or a safety

The correct way to clean the nose is to press one nostril closed at a time with your fingers; and open your mouth as you exhale to "blow" out excess mucous, etc. from the opposite nostril. This will prevent pressure from affecting the ears or sinuses.

Chapter 7

ACCOMPANIMENT AND EQUIPMENT RESOURCES

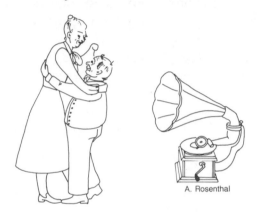

A. Rosenthal

CRITERIA FOR SELECTION

Music for Accompanying Exercise and Creative Activities

We have found that a varied selection of long-playing recordings and a simple collection of rhythm instruments are the ideal accompaniment resources for the geriatric dance/movement program.

Cassettes or reel-to-reel tapes are not very convenient to use during therapeutic dance sessions. It is difficult to find the exact selection on a tape and attempting to repeat or to change music may necessitate lengthy rewinding and adjustments at the tape machine.

is usually preferable to work without live musical accompaniment if the person or accompanist has not experienced with a therapeutic group. Also it is essential for the leader and the accompanist to work and plan together so that there is a unified approach to the program. Sometimes the session becomes entertainment or performance rather than a participation therapeutic activity because there is limited interaction among the leader, group, and accompanist.

When musical recordings are used there is a great deal of freedom of selection and flexibility in length, volume, and pace of the accompaniment. The most convenient phonograph records are those that have fairly long bands of one-and-a-half to three-minute duration. In order to encourage constructive recall it is also desirable to include familiar melodies from folk music, semiclassical, and popular tunes of the 1920s, 1930s, and 1940s. Simple (not overwhelmingly symphonic versions) of classical and contemporary concert selections with varied tonal qualities are helpful for creative expression. It is also good to choose music that reflects the nationality or ethnicity of the group members.

Many nursing homes and senior citizens facilities have music collections that are used by the music therapist or the social activities personnel. These may include folk songs and popular tunes that will add to the enjoyment of the dance exercise sessions.

Characteristics of Appropriate Rhythm Instruments

Percussion instruments that are primarily rhythmic rather than melodic are the most versatile equipment for geriatric groups. They are simple to use, safe to handle, and they produce immediate individual and group response. If the emphasis is placed on the physical action and the group interaction involved in playing, then rhythm band instruments offer great enjoyment and challenge to the older adult.

Portable instruments are ideal so that the leader-therapist can move around the group while playing. Size and weight are important considerations also, so that the participants can easily hold and manipulate them. Over the years, we have found that the most popular instruments among residents and participants in geriatric movement sessions, are the maraccas and tambourines. We have learned that it is worthwhile to purchase sturdily constructed drums and tambourines, and professionally made maraccas and cymbals, rather than toys, in order to enjoy good tone and longer, safer use. It is possible, however, to construct inexpensive, colorful percussion instruments. Rattles, rhythm sticks, and drums can be made from everyday objects like plastic and metal containers, beans, buttons, Christmas bells, thread spindles, cardboard rolls, and even tableware. A source for descriptions and instructions to make instruments is Gladys A. Fleming's book, *Creative Rhythmic Movement* (36).

Rhythm instruments may be used by the leader-therapist to establish a pulse or beat for group activity and to inspire movement. Or they may be played by group members for individual or ensemble music.

The quantity and variety of an instrument collection will depend on the size and the interests of the group. It is suggested that enough choice and challenge be available to fulfill the therapeutic possibilities of improving hand function and providing opportunities for group stimulation.

LISTS OF SUGGESTED MUSIC

For Opening and Closing of Sessions

Bright, rousing strongly rhythmic selections that inspire hand clapping and foot tapping are good for beginning a session. Many groups enjoy starting the activity with an adapted dance pattern that involves greeting the members.

... soothing, soothing, soothing, moderately paced music that inspires ... and group ... ...deal. Melodies help members sway and stretch while feeling good about saying farewell until the next time.

Sometimes a tune can become almost a ritual and be used at each meeting of the group. For example, Jewish music could ... often enjoy "Shalom Alichem" played for both opening and closing of the dance/movement session.

Opening:

"Happy Days Are Here Again"
"The Happy Wanderer"
"Do Re Me" from "The Sound of Music"
"Alexander's Ragtime Band"
"Seventy-Six Trombones"
"Getting To Know You" from "The King and I"
"Bingo" (see page134) for greeting dance
"Consider Yourself At Home" (see page 143 for greet-
    ing dance)
"Funiculi Funicula"

Closing:

"So Long, It's Been Good To Know You"
"Aloha Oe"
"When You're Smiling"
"Auld Lang Syne"
"Goodnight Irene"
"Goodnight Sweetheart"
"After the Ball Is Over"
"I Could Have Danced All Night"
"I'll See You Again"
"Always"

For Exercise Accompaniment

It is often helpful to sustain interest and unify the group with well-selected music. We find that moderately paced melodies of 3/4 or 4/4 time are most appropriate. The older adults appreciate melodies that they recognize and phrasing they can anticipate.

> "Cruising Down the River"
> "Let Me Call You Sweetheart"
> "Orchids in the Moonlight"
> "Syncopated Clock"
> "Hernando's Hideaway"
> "The Spanish Flea"
> "Glow Worm"
> "Java"
> "March of the Siamese Children"
> "This Old Man"
> "Colonel Bogey March"

Also see pages 229, 230, and 231 for additional music that we have enjoyed using with geriatric groups.

LIST OF SUGGESTED RHYTHM INSTRUMENTS & MUSICAL COLLECTIONS

Rhythm Instruments

DRUMS

1. Bongo drums
2. African tomba drum (Figure 7–1)
3. Wigman hand drum

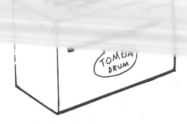

Figure 7-1   African tomba drum. Kassoy

4. Israeli or Turkish drum (dumbek) (Figure 7–2)
5. Oriental hand drum (Figure 7–3)

RATTLES AND BELLS

1. Maraccas
2. Tambourines (small or medium size)
3. Headless tambourines
4. Handle bells (Figure 7–4)
5. Bracelet bells (Figure 7–5)
6. Stick bells

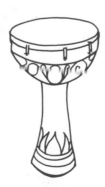

Figure 7-2   Israeli hand drum. Kassoy

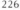

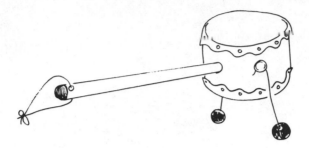

Figure 7-3   Oriental hand drum. Kassoy

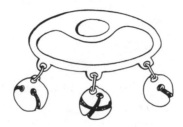

Figure 7-4   Handle bells. Kassoy

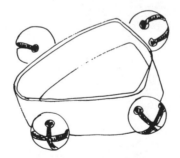

Figure 7-5   Bracelet bells. Kassoy

CLAPPERS AND CLAVES

1. Stick castanets
2. Elastic castanets
3. Rhythm sticks
4. Temple blocks (Figure 7–6)
5. Wooden tone blocks

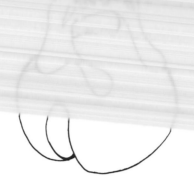

Figure 7-6   Temple block. Kassoy

1. Finger cymbals (zills) (Figure 7–7)
2. Cymbals
3. Triangles
4. Gong

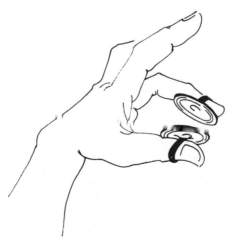

Figure 7-7   Finger cymbals. Kassoy

RATCHETS

1. Latin scraper (*guarira*) (Figure 7–8)
2. Sand blocks

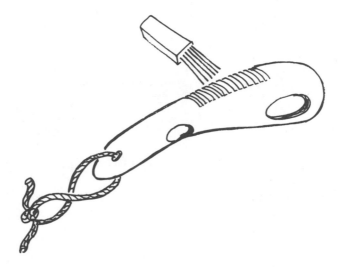

Figure 7-8   Latin scraper (*guarira*). Kassoy

Recorded Collections of Music

These are offered to indicate the type and variety of useful musical recordings. Many of the selections have been recorded by numerous artists and different companies, so that this list may serve only as a guide to personal selections at local music outlets.

"The Brahms I Love by
   Artur Rubinstein"   RCA LSC 3186
"My Favorite Chopin by
   Van Cliburn"   RCA LSC 7078
"Debussy Greatest Hits"   Columbia MS 7883
"The French Album"   RCA LSC ...

"Grieg Collection"   Angel ...
"The Great Victor
   Herbert"   London SPC 21143
"Itzhak Perlman Plays Fritz
   Kreisler"   Angel S-37171
"The Mozart Album"   Columbia MG 30841
"Johann Strauss
   Collection"   Columbia M 34125
"Tschaikowsky Ballet
   Album"   Columbia MG 30297

ETHNIC

"Dance Along With Mitch
   —Latin Style"   Hoctor HLP 3083
"Spirituals from Tuskegee
   Institute"   Westminster WES 8154
"Oh Glory Hallelujah—
   Bessie Griffen"   Columbia, Epic BN 26101
"Bar Mitzvah Favorites"   Fiesta FLPS 1590
"Mandolins In Italy"   Fiesta FLPS 1750
"Irish Dance Party"   Avoca 33 ST 101
"This Is Our Scotland"   Fiesta FLPS 1603
"Syrtaki Bouzouki Music"   London SPW 1003
"Polish Songs and
   Dances"   Fiesta FLPS 1791
"Drums of Passion—
   Olatunji"   Columbia CG 33654

"Russian Folklore in Song & Dance"	Fiesta FLPS 1709
"Twenty Great Gospel Songs"	Gusto PO 292
"Salute To Israel"	Monitor MFS 746
"Israeli Folk Dance Medley"	Tikva LPT 106

POPULAR

"George M. Cohan— Yankee Doodle Dandy"	Olympic Olr 7111
"The Best of Tommy Dorsey"	RCA ANLI 1087
"The Eddie Duchin Story"	Columbia C 59420
"Duke Ellington's Jazz Party"	Columbia JCS 8127
"American Colleges Sing Stephen Foster"	Request SRLP 8028
"Encore Collection— George Gershwin"	Columbia EN 2 13719
"Sixteen Classical Rags of Scott Joplin"	RCA ARLI 1257
"Let's Keep Dancing to the All Time Golden Favorites"	Thunderbird TH 5
"Liberace Candlelight Series"	American Variety Int'l AVL 1023
"The Best of Guy Lombardo"	Decca DX 5B 7185
"Glenn Miller Parade of Hits"	Camden ACL 7009
"An Enchanted Evening With Mantovani"	London LL 766
"Columbia Album of Richard Rodgers"	Columbia En 2 13725

SPECIAL

"All Purpose Folk Dances —Michael Herman Orchestra"	RCA EPA 4138
"All Time Favorite Waltzes"	Hoctor Records, Vol I—HLP 4077; Vol II—HLP 4070
"Arthur Fiedler Collection of Favorites"	RCA CRL I—2064
"The Roaring 20's—16 Greatest Hits—Enoch Light"	ABC 746
"Songs of Many Cultures"	Educational Activities KEA 1139
"Special Music for Special People"	Educational Activities AR85
"A Treasury of Great American Favorites"	RCA ARL 2—1421
"Twenty Stereo Spectaculars"	RCA CRL 3—0985
"Wake Up, Calm Down"	Educational Activities Vol. I—AR 695 Vol. II—AR 699
"The Whole World Dances —Geula Gill"	Elektra EKS 7206

List of Objects and Equipment

A successful therapist is alert to the creative possibilities of objects from many sources. There are unlimited uses for the following found and collected items.

Balls—beach, nerf (sponge), fabric, styrofoam or whiffle (string, ribbon or elastic can be attached)

Balloons—(strings, ribbon or elastic should be attached)

Boxes—cardboard, clean waste paper baskets

Contact paper and tinfoil

Elastic—rope, webbing

Fabric—velvet, satin, nubby tweeds

Fans—paper, folding wood or plastic

Feathers—duster with handle, single ostrich or peacock

Flashlights—lighweight, small

Flowers—fabric, tissue paper

Frisbees—plastic discs, approximately 9 inches in diameter

Gloves or mittens

Hats—cloth or paper

Hoops—lightweight plastic, approximately 15 inches in diameter

Paper—streamers, plates (plastic coated), cardboard tubes from paper towel or tinfoil

Ribbons—lightweight plastic or cloth

Scarves—chiffon or silk—approximately 20 inches square

Sticks—shortened broomsticks, canes, dowels, wands, batons, or rods (streamers or scarves may be attached)

String—yarn or clothesline

Sam Ash
178 Mamaroneck Avenue
White Plains, New York 10600

Canadian F.D.S. Audio Visual Aids
605 King Street W.
Toronto, Ontario

Herbet Dancewear
902 Broadway
New York, New York 10010

House of Musical Instruments
305 South Washington Street
Berkeley Springs, West Virginia 25411

Peripole Music Co.
Browns Mills, New Jersey 08015

Charles Ponte Music Co.
142 West 46 Street
New York, New York 10036

Record Center
1614 North Pulaski
Chicago, Illinois 60639

Sandy's Sounds
20 Ronald Drive
Monsey, New York 10952

Dance Etc.
5897 College Avenue
Oakland, California 91610

Distributors of Dance Books and Recordings

Stanley Bowmar Co. Inc.
4 Broadway
Valhalla, New York 10595

Breglio's School Supplies
219-10 Hillside Ave.
Queens Village, Queens, New York 11427

Bridges Dance Wear
310 West Jefferson
Dallas, Texas 75208

Children's Music Center, Inc.
5373 West Pico Blvd.
Los Angeles, California 90019

Dance Record Distributors
Children's Record Guild, Young People's Records,
Folkraft Records
1159 Broad Street
Newark, New Jersey 07114

Educational Activities, Inc.
1937 North Grand Ave.
Baldwin, New York 11510

Educational Record Sales
157 Chambers Street
New York, New York 10007

Festival Folk Shop
2769 West Pico Blvd.
Los Angeles, California 90006

Gateway Record Shop
10013 N.E. Wasco
Portland, Oregon 97220

Sam Goody
Green Acres Shopping Center
Valley Stream, New York 11580
(Sam Goody has several stores in the New York
Metropolitan area)

Herbet Dancewear
902 Broadway
New York, New York 10010

Hoctor Records
Waldwick, New Jersey 07463

Kimbo Educational Records
P.O. Box 246
Deal, New Jersey 07723

Koxana
3022 S. Washington St.
Seattle, Washington 98144

Ed Kremer's Folk Shop
161 Turk Street
San Francisco, California 94102

A.B. Le Crone Rhythms Record Co.
819 N.W. 92 Street
Oklahoma City, Oklahoma 73114

Lyons
530 Riverview Avenue
Elkhart, Indiana 46514

Phil Maran's Folk Shop
1531 Clay Street
Oakland, California 94612

Petrella's Record Shop
2014 W. Darby Road
Mavertown, Pennsylvania 19083

Plays, Inc.
8 Arlington Street
Boston, Massachusetts 02116

Q T Records
Statler Record Corporation
73 Fifth Avenue
New York, New York 10003

Randolph Associates, Inc.
1231 Race Street
Philadelphia, Pennsylvania 19107

Record Center
1614 North Pulaski
Chicago, Illinois 60639

Record Hunter
507 Fifth Avenue
New York, New York 10017

Rhythms Production Records
Whitney Building
Box 34485
Los Angeles, California 90034

Sets In Order
462 North Robertson Blvd.
Los Angeles, California 90048

Washington Records
1319 F Street in Avenue NW
Washington, D.C. 20030

World Tone Music
160 West 48 Avenue
New York, New York 10011

Chapter 8

EVALUATION AND JUSTIFICATION OF PROGRAM

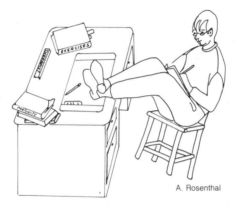

A. Rosenthal

PURPOSES OF RECORD KEEPING

Most programs require reports or record keeping in order to justify their existence and support. The activities specialist will also be able to benefit personally and professionally from the collection of anecdotal or questionnaire-type evaluations. Assessment of the abilities and progress of group members is used to develop the dance/movement program. Leaders will find that it is possible to select appropriate activities and to gauge the effectiveness of their efforts by utilizing information that is gained from these reports. We have found that written records of sessions, with references to specific individual responses, are also very helpful to clarify our work. An authority in the field of therapeutic

PROBLEMS OF EVALUATION

Evaluation, although valuable, is time consuming and often difficult to accomplish for large numbers of participants with patterns of brief continuity. Most geriatric programs have problems of sporadic attendance, large-size groups, and administrative constraints. In addition, part-time movement specialists may find record keeping and staff consultation especially difficult if the full-time staff is not available for conferences or is only minimally interested in the progress of dance/movement sessions. It is certainly very helpful to be able to discuss the overall program and your experiences with the activities director, the center administrator, or the person in charge of patient services. Also, inviting medical and social work personnel to observe sessions will often result in new allies or advisors. We have had success in enlisting the support of our colleagues by sharing brief accounts or comments that come out of sessions through the in-house paper or newsletter. Another rewarding project has been to schedule staff workshops and participation-discussion sessions for colleagues.

A long-standing problem that has plagued the field of dance therapy and many of the other arts activities, has been sparse and unvalidated research. There is a lack of creditable testing methods and standards of evaluation for emotional and psychological responses. Most scientific research techniques do not seem to be readily applicable to therapeutic dance/movement. Our goals are qualitative rather than quantitative. We count ourselves successful when our work produces a smile, a renewed interest in the present, or a small reduction of pain or discomfort. Measurements of the range of motion for each body joint or assessment of physical fitness parameters such as cardiorespiratory efficiency are helpful to gauge an individual's physical potential or improvement, but they do not reveal the mental, emotional, and social changes brought about through dance/movement sessions. Also, as practicing clinical dance therapist, Elizabeth Rosen has mentioned in her book, *Dance in Psychotherapy,* the forces contributing to behavior changes can rarely be isolated (38).

We believe that the subjective judgment of an experienced and perceptive person can be accurately descriptive of the benefits that result from therapeutic movement. Therefore, we use the questionnaire technique to elicit responses from professional staff and participants of the program. We also welcome written reports and comments from trained observers or leaders. This information has not been tabulated or cited statistically, but it does provide an in-depth picture of the accomplishment and limitations of the activity. These evaluations can be viewed as valuable additions to the clinical record.

ANECDOTAL RECORDS

Written notes or outlines of sessions that include references to particularly successful or disappointing occurrences can be made by the leader-therapist, a colleague or staff member, or even by a group member. We find that sometimes a special choice of music or a certain way of presenting a movement activity will provide the impetus for positive change. Noting this in a log gives the leader-therapist an opportunity to acknowledge its significance and perhaps find ways to build on this and share it with other staff members.

she let her hands on_
ered her ears at the fourth session, I was
she asked in a very low voice, "Was the last dance we did an
Israeli or a Greek Dance?" I told her she was a good judge
of music and dance; it was Greek. She has been participating
more since then. (Check with the social worker for ethnic
roots.)

Mr. C. is in good physical condition, but partially disoriented. At first he showed no interest or reaction to the
session. He sat and stared. Every few minutes he would leave
his seat and walk around the room asking for a cigarette and
return to his chair. I played "Anniversary Waltz." He
grabbed me, held me tightly in dance position, sang the tune
loudly with "La, la, la . . .," and waltzed me vigorously but
gracefully around the room. For the next three sessions he
participated in the folk dances and we regularly danced together to "Anniversary Waltz." Then he would resume his
begging for cigarettes. There have now been 17 sessions
and he has become an active participant for almost the entire
session and only rarely stops to ask for cigarettes.

Mrs. A., in her eighties with one leg in a cast, walks with
a walker. I played selections from "Tschaikowsky Ballet Album" and she extended the encased leg forward and raised
the arm on the same side overhead in a fairly accurate sem-
blance of a balletic position. I complimented her and the
group expressed appreciation. She told us that her sister had
been a ballet dancer and that this was the first time it felt
good to remember and good for her to try to dance. (We will
try more classical music; note to psychologist about her family.)

Mrs. G. is a diabetic who has had both legs amputated.
She has been depressed and withdrawn and has participated
minimally in the sessions. I distributed a cardboard tube
with attached plastic streamers to each group member. We

moved them in various ways in time to musical accompaniment. Suddenly Mrs. A. said with a smile on her face, "Look
what I can do!" She had found her own way of using the
"wand" and the entire group began imitating her movement. She was delighted with her achievement and with its
acceptance by the group.

Another double leg amputee, Mr. Z., came to the first
session and placed himself and his wheelchair at the far end
of the room, separating himself from the others. When the
music started his face became animated. He observed the
session. At the closing, I went around the room saying goodbye to each person. I shook hands with him and he said,
"God bless you." The next week I asked him to come closer
to the group, but he refused. He did participate in some of
the activity and particularly enjoyed playing a maracca in
time to the music. He smiled continuously. I asked after a
few more sessions why he didn't come closer to the rest of
the group. He said, "I have no legs. I can't dance. I'd rather
stay in the back." I answered him, "Dancing is feeling the
music inside of you and moving in your own special way."
He seemed pleased and moved his chair a little closer. He
joined our circle the next time and felt quite at ease.

Another type of narrative record keeping that is useful
for assessing the effectiveness of one's work is the tran-
scribing of participants' comments and responses. The following excerpts from letters and remarks are examples that
we treasure. We have utilized them to develop our skills
and encourage support from our colleagues.

Specific Remarks and Quotations

Mr. K., aged 85, told us this as an illustration of his pride in
his participation in the movement sessions: "My son was so
surprised that I exercise every week. He didn't know that
there were special programs for people my age. It certainly
made me feel good to tell him that I'm not too old to be
active!"

Another octagenarian said, "My husband and my children can't believe what I'm now able to do."

ment sessions are comm...
now than I did when I came in today.   You lo...
20 years younger!" "I wouldn't miss our weekly sessions; it's
like going to a party."

A 99-year-old woman resident of a nursing home comes
over to the leader at the end of each session to say thank you
and to make certain that we have an appointment for the
following week.

Mr. C. is a stroke victim with aphasia and says only one
word clearly "Wunderbar." It's possible to tell how much
he is enjoying the session by the emphasis he gives to that
word.

The reactivation of pleasant memories was attested to
by Mrs. T. who said, "We used to do movements like this
when I was a girl in Germany taking rhythmic gymnastics in
school. Ach, those were good times."

This poem is an example of the many tributes from
loyal group members:

Sonya is our teacher, and boy how she does teach,
She has us stretching every way, as far as we can reach.
The exercises that we do are really very good,
She always stresses breathing, the way each person
    should.
We go around the clock using only our eyes, to
    strengthen them by exercise.
And when we do the Japanese dance, we have to wipe
    our brow,
The movements are really graceful, but we get
    through it somehow.

Then comes meditation time, as we quietly sit and
   rest,
With the music softly playing, I think that I like this
   best.
And when the session is over, I feel a little sad,
But then I think of the following week, and once again
   I'm glad.
P.S. I also enjoy hearing Sonya laugh, I'm glad she is
   on our teacher staff.

                                 written by Alex Markoff, aged 77.

ABILITY ASSESSMENTS

Another good way to discover the need or value of various
elements in the dance/movement program is to rate the
abilities of participants at the beginning of an activities
program and then again after a specified length of time.
Helene Lefco, dance therapist, in her book, *Dance Therapy*,
gives an additional reason for determining the physical
capabilities of clients. She says, "Because mental health
depends in part upon the body's muscular ability to stay
flexible and pliable, the dance therapist must first evaluate
the areas of rigidity in her patients" (39). The frequency of
the sessions and the regularity of the individual's attendance must be noted, in addition to pertinent facts about
the person's age and medical restrictions. The ability as-
sessments must also be evaluated with some attention to
the amount of physical therapy the patient is getting in
addition to the dance/movement program.

   Assessment of the client's capabilities can be done
ideally with one to three people at a time. If larger groups
of clients are evaluated at the same time, then only a brief
visual judgment can be made using as many of the catego-
ries in the following listing as possible. The abilities listed
in the evaluation form include physical range of movement.

members as they attempt each activity. The measures
(S—Strong, M—Moderate, W—Weak, or N—Nonperformance) are subjective and will be given by comparison to
the performance of an average person of the same age. For
example, an 80-year-old nursing home resident who performs an activity at the same level as an average, active
80-year-old would be given an "S" on the rating form.
Obviously the interpretation of this rating scale will be
significant primarily for the person doing the testing.

The importance of the results, to us, lies in the record
of change from the first evaluation to the second evaluation. The ratings are compared only with the individual's
own scores and not to those of other group members. Our
results show that slight to marked improvements in the
range of movement of the torso and upper limbs are seen
in almost all clients in health related facilities and golden
age groups. The areas of rhythmic and creative response
also indicate postitive change after consistent participation.
Lower limb mobility and space orientation, however, does
not seem to improve as dramatically with the geriatric
groups we tested.

Evaluation of Dance/Movement Capabilities

CLIENT'S NAME ———————— —— AGENCY ————————

AGE ——— Confined to chair: All the time/Part of time/Not necessary
Able to walk: Unaided/With Cane/With Walker

MEDICAL ASSESSMENT ——————————————————————

Abilities are rate:		Dates Administered:	
S – Strong performance		1st	,19
M – Moderate performance			
W – Weak performance			
N – Nonperformance		2nd	,19

ATTENDANCE: (Check below each time client attends session.)

___/_/_/_/_/_/_/_/_/_/_/_/_/_/ TOTAL #___ sessions

(Place an S, M, W, or N in the appropriate column to signify the performance level for right or left side.)

	1st Eval.		2nd Eval.	
	Right	Left	Right	Left
Raise both shoulders and lower				
Alternately raise each shoulder and lower				
Bring both shoulders forward and backward				
Circle both shoulders toward the back				
Place hands on shoulders with elbows foward				
Place hands on head				
Extended hands over head				
Circle hands from wrist				
Circle extended arms at sides, upward, and back				
Alternately lift one knee and replace				
Extend both legs straight forward				
Alternately circle foot, keep contact with floor				

(Place a check in the appropriate box.)

	1st Eval.				2nd Eval.			
	S	M	W	N	S	M	W	N
Head and neck mobility:								
Upward								
Downward								
To left side								
To right side								
Circling								
Breathing ease:								
Inhaling								
Exhaling								
Movement coordination								
Rhythmic response								
Creative response								
Space Orientation:								
Range-Size (does large and small movement)								
Directionality (moves fwd. bkwd.swd. diag. circ.)								
Level (moves from lying to sitting to stand)								

	1st Eval.				2nd Eval.			
Energy use: (Check applicable box)								
Bound (tense)								
Free (relaxed)								
Direct (focused)								
Indirect (flexible)								
Light								
Heavy								

QUESTIONNAIRES TO DETERMINE PARTICIPANT RESPONSE

Brief questions or opportunities to check off specific changes that have been noticed can be presented to group members or staff. We have made up simple questionnaires and given them to our clients in senior citizens centers. We have also asked geriatrics personnel such as physicians, social workers, supervisory nurses, and activities directors to evaluate the response of individual clients to the therapeutic movement sessions. Since we did not attempt to assemble large numbers of responses nor did we identify specific data for each respondent or group, our tabulations are not for statistical purposes. We have tried to determine a consensus or an overall reaction regarding the value of the activity for the client. We also prepared and circulated an evaluation form for staff members to note their more general comments about the dance/movement program and its effect on the specific population as a whole. Copies of the questionnaires we have utilized are on pages 250 and 251.

Results of Questionnaires Answered by Staff Members

The staff evaluation of a six-month program with weekly movement sessions involving patients ranging in age from 74 to 92 years old at the Jewish Institute for Geriatric Care in New Hyde Park, Long Island produced the following comments. Three professional staff members answered separate, detailed questionnaires (page 255) concerning the participation of individual patients. Without exception, the staff observed positive changes in all of the patients' behavior after therapeutic movement sessions. They overwhelmingly stated that the patients looked forward to the weekly sessions. The changes most often cited by the trained staff members (a physician, a social worker, and a supervisory nurse) were improved self-image and better concentration. Other frequently noted benefits included alertness and the alleviation of anxiety symptoms.

mental-emotional levels, all look forward eagerly to the
weekly sessions. In a heterogeneous group of blind and
sighted elderly, ranging in age from the late sixties to 90
years old, the group worker found that the experience for
the blind members ". . . seems to have made liberated hu-
mans out of them." She stated that she had "not seen them
enter into anything else that gives them so much joy." Also
she noted that one man had shown an increase in strength
and a marked improvement in the ease and speed of his
walking. The volunteer leaders of a Jewish day center
group wrote enthusiastic evaluations of the weekly dance
therapy sessions attended by 30 to 35 persons between 70
and 96 years of age. The participants are predominantly
female and they are delighted with the opportunity to socialize, practice therapeutic exercises, and learn ethnic
dances. At the Jewish Home and Hospital for the Aged in
New York City and the Jewish Institute for Geriatric Care
in New Hyde Park, New York, supervisory personnel were
unanimous in their praise for the dance/movement sessions. They wrote of the patients' anticipation of the sessions and the regularity with which relatively healthy,
disabled, and even disoriented patients enthusiastically attended. Both groups are comprised of more females than
males from predominantly German and Russian Jewish
backgrounds. They enjoy the music and the expressive-
creative activity. For a few of the patients, this is the only
group offering in which they participate.

Staff Evaluation of Participant Response to Geriatric Movement Sessions

STAFF MEMBER Name: _____ Date: _____

PATIENT Name: _____ Age: _____ General Condition _____

1. Does client look forward to the movement sessions?
   YES _____   NO _____

2. Have you noticed positive changes in the client's behavior after dance/movement sessions?   YES _____   NO _____

   (If YES)   A. Physical Changes
   Improvement of: (a) appetite _____
                     (b) sleeping habits _____
                     (c) bladder control _____
                     (d) flexibility—mobility _____
                     (e) coordination _____
                     (f) muscle strength _____
                     (g) posture _____

   B. Emotional–Mental Changes
   Alleviation of: (a) anxiety symptoms _____
                      (b) attention demands _____
   Improvement of: (c) self–image _____
                      (d) memory _____
                      (e) concentration _____
                      (f) alertness _____

   C. Social Changes
   Improvement in attitude toward:
                      (a) staff _____
                      (b) other patients _____
                      (c) family _____

Additional Comments _____

_____

_____

~~STAFF EVALUATION OF THERAPEUTIC DANCE/MOVEMENT~~
~~PROGRAM~~

~~NAME OF STAFF MEMBER~~ ~~DATE~~

~~POSITION~~ ~~NAME OF AGENCY~~

~~1. Do the clients look forward to the therapeutic movement sessions?~~

~~YES~~ ~~NO~~

2. Have you noticed positive changes in the participants' behavior after dance/movement sessions?

YES _____   NO _____

ADDITIONAL COMMENTS: (Specific details regarding clients and/or their responses to the therapeutic dance program, such as the following—age range, physical condition, mental–emotional status, ethnic background, sex, socio–economic position, etc.)

_____

_____

_____

_____

_____

_____

_____

_____

_____

_____

_____

_____

_____

_____

251

Results of Questionnaires Answered by Clients

The responses of day care senior citizen center participants to a questionnaire about their dance/movement sessions gave us some information about their preferences for certain activities. We also found that the questions presented an opportunity for the older adults to analyze and verbalize some of their feelings and reactions to the group and their participation in it. In addition, the questionnaire served as a way for them to consciously assess their achievements and give recognition to their needs.

A questionnaire, such as this one (page 255), is necessarily limited or biased by the selection of choices offered and by the range of comprehension and objectivity of the respondent. We found it helpful to allow enough time for explaining the questions and encouraging the group to be as careful and accurate as they could be when answering. It was not feasible for us to give the questionnaire to patients in skilled, long-term nursing facilities. We believe that the limitations of hearing, sight, and comprehension, plus the physical difficulties of recording the answers, outweigh the values that might be gained from such survey results. We would recommend individual interviews with therapeutic dance/movement participants in nursing homes and hospitals. During this time questions such as those we have used might be asked.

The questionnaire results from the members of three geriatric day centers with groups of 14, 15, and 21 people, respectively (50 in total), supplied us with a unanimous "YES" to "Do you feel better after you join in our sessions?" We conclude that this is an important factor in the interest and dedication of the 46 who attended weekly sessions on a regular basis. The results of the questionnaire indicated that, within a continuity range of one month to four years, the majority of those queried had been participating for two months (21 persons) or seven months (16 persons).

From one person said that the exercises helped them relax at appropriate periods and that they often practiced such as the dance exercises on their own at home. At least one piece of evidence of the dance/movement activities was apparent to all but five of the people answering the questionnaire. Twenty-four (almost half) of the women and men found it easier to sleep, 27 noted improved ability to relax, and 28 said others that deep breathing was easier for them since joining the movement program.

The emotional benefits that were most frequently noted by 48 of the group of 50 tabulated were feeling: "more cheerful" (30), "less tense" (24), and "more self-assured" (21). Of interest to us were the 15 people who mentioned that they felt more enthusiastic and an equal number who felt more tired because of our sessions. We attach more significance to the 41 older adults who believe that their powers of concentration and mental involvement have improved because of the dance therapy sessions. (One member of the group did not notice any improvement and eight people did not answer this question.)

The friendly group atmosphere was attested to by almost every respondent (49). And the individual's more outgoing enjoyment of new personal contacts was noted by 42 persons in contrast to three who noted no change in their social attitudes and five who did not answer that question.

We found question 9, "What part of the session do you enjoy the most? (indicate one)," difficult to tabulate because many of the clients circled more than one choice, a few circled all of them, and some circled only one. Exercise and breathing and relaxation activities are the easiest to present and therefore are very successful with comparatively large therapeutic groups. Other aspects, such as massage, are very well received and might be rated most enjoyable if they could be included more often. But they require a one-to-one relationship and more time for organization. The results of our questionnaire show that exactly half of the clients (25) said that the exercises were the part of the session they enjoyed most; the same number (13 each) preferred the music and dance portions and the breathing and relaxation parts. Five (10 percent) enjoyed the massage most, and four (8 percent) found the health suggestions most enjoyable.

RECOMMENDATIONS FOR FUTURE EVALUATION

The field of therapeutic dance will be ideally served by more refined techniques of research and analysis. We hope that behavioral scientists and researchers in the areas of therapeutic modalities will direct their efforts toward the assessment of dance/movement programs for the aged.

Perhaps more controlled populations, consistent personnel doing the evaluations, and improved assessment techniques are what is needed. In addition, the construction of validated test instruments for geriatric populations, similar to the Oseretsky Tests of Motor Proficiency (40), would be of great benefit. Also the compilation of movement observation studies by effort/shape specialists can have positive value.

We look forward to improved geriatric dance/movement that is a result of better programming content and evaluation.

3. Do you also try to do these exercises on your own?   YES   NO

4. Since joining our sessions, have you found it easier to:

sleep   relax   breathe deeply   walk   write

bend   climb stairs   stand on your feet   sit   sew

EMOTIONAL-MENTAL BENEFITS

5. Did our sessions make you feel:

less tense   less lonely   more cheerful

more optimistic   more tense   more tired

less anxious   more self-assured   more confused

more enthusiastic

6. Did you find that your powers of concentration or mental involvement improved because of our sessions?   YES   NO

SOCIAL BENEFITS

7. Did you feel that the sessions produced a friendly atmosphere with
   the people in the group?   YES   NO

8. Did you become more outgoing and enjoy new personal contacts?

                                                       YES   NO

9. What part of the session do you enjoy the most? (indicate <u>ONE</u>)

   exercises   breathing and relaxation   massage

   health suggestions   music and dance

10. I have attended dance sessions: REGULARLY   IRREGULARLY

   for   ONE month   TWO months   THREE months

         FOUR months   FIVE months   SIX months

         SEVEN months   ONE YEAR   TWO YEARS

CHAPTER 1

1. A look at Americans in the year 2000. *U.S. News and World Report,* March 1935, P. 35.

2. Martin, W. C. (Ed.) *Aging and total health.* St. Petersburg, Fla. Eckerd College Gerontology Center, 1976. P. 147.

3. *The New York Times,* June 19, 1977, Section E. P. 9.

4. *Great Neck Record,* August 5, 1976. P. 12A.

5. Pitt, B. *Psychogeriatrics.* London: Churchill-Livingstone, 1974. P. 136.

6. Brown, L., & Ellis, E. D. (Eds.) *The later years.* Littleton, Mass.: Publishing Sciences Group, Inc., 1974.

7. Jeffers, F. C. You and the aging in your community. *The Gerontologist,* 1970, **10,** 57–59.

8. Lindsey, R. Los Angeles News Bureau Chief, *The N.Y. Times* Medical Column, June 19, 1977.

9. Inceni, A. G. *Winds of change: A report of a conference on activity programs in long-term care institutions.* Chicago, Ill.: A.H.A., 1971. P. 26.

10. Galton, L. *Don't give up on an aging parent.* New York: Crown Publishers, 1975. P. 167.

11. Schilder, P. *The image and appearance of the human body.* England: Routledge & Kegan Paul, 1925. P. 112.

12. Helm, J. B., & Gill, K. L. An essential resource for the aging; Dance therapy. *Dance Research Journal of CORD,* Fall–Winter 1974–5, **Vii:I,** P. 4.

13. Brunner, D., & Jokl, E. (Eds.) *Physical activity and aging.* Vol. 4. Baltimore, Md.: University Park Press, 1970. P. 302.

14. deVries, H. A. Education for physical fitness in the later years. In Grabowski, S., Mason, (W.), (Eds.) *Learning for aging.* Washington, D.C.: Adult Education Assn., 1974. P. 250–267.

15. Op. cit.

16. Bright, R. *Music in geriatric care.* New York: St. Martin's Press, 1972. P. 31.

17. Pitt, B. *Psychogeriatrics.* P. 146. London: Churchill-Livingstone, 1974.

18. Schwartz, C. G. Rehabilitation of mental hospital patients, *Public Health Monograph* 1953, No. 17, U.S. Dept. of H.E.W., Wash., D.C. Rosen, E. *Dance in psychotherapy.* New York: Dance Horizons Republication, 1974. P. 19.

19. Klopfer, W. G. Psychological stresses of old age. *Geriatrics,* 1958, **13,** 529–531.

20. Salkin, J. *Body-ego technique.* Springfield, Ill.: Charles C Thomas, 1973. P. 52.

21. Hirschberg, G., Lewis, L., & Thomas, D. *Rehabilitation.* Philadelphia: Lippincott, 1964.

CHAPTER 3

22. Salkin, J. *Body-ego technique.* Springfield, Ill.: Charles C. Thomas, 1973. P. 9.

CHAPTER 4

23. Kraus, H. *Principles and practice of therapeutic exercises.* Springfield, Ill.: Charles C. Thomas, 1963. P. xi.

CHAPTER 5

27. Harris, J., Pittman, A., & Waller, M. *Dance awhile*. (5th ed.) Minneapolis, Minn.: Burgess Publishing Co., 1978.
    Hayes, E. R. *An introduction to the teaching of dance*. New York: Ronald Press Co., 1964. P. 241–289.

28. Bright, R. *Music in geriatric care*. New York: St. Martin's Press, 1972. P. 90.

29. Merritt, M. *Dance therapy programs for nursing homes*. (Rev. ed.) Boston, Mass.: Unitarian Universalist Assn., 1971.

30. Bright, R. *Music in geriatric care*, New York: St. Martin's Press, 1972. P. 31.

31. Boxburger, R., & Cotter, V. W. The geriatric patient. In E. G. Thayer (Ed.) *Music in therapy*. New York: Macmillan Co., 1968. P. 271.

CHAPTER 6

32. Pitt, B. *Psychogeriatrics*, page 117. London: Churchill-Livingstone, 1974.

33. Kraus, H. *Principles and practice of therapeutic exercises*. Springfield, Ill.: Charles C. Thomas, 1956. P. vii.

34. Davis, J. C. Team management of Parkinson's disease. *Journal of Occupational Therapy*, May–June 1977, **31**:5 P. 300.

35. President's Council on Fitness & Sports & the Administration on Aging. *The fitness challenge in the later years*. Wash., D.C.: Administration on Aging Pub. #802, May 1968.

CHAPTER 7

36. Fleming, G. A. *Creative rhythmic movement* New Jersey: Prentice-Hall Inc., 1976. P. 247-263.

CHAPTER 8

37. Mosey, C. *Activities therapy* New York: Raven Press Publishers, 1973. P. 83.

38. Rosen, E. *Dance in psychotherapy.* New York: Dance Horizons Republication, 1974.

39. Lefco, H. *Dance therapy.* Chicago: Nelson Hall, 1973. P. 132.

40. Doll, E. A. ed. *Oseretsky Tests of Motor Proficiency.* Circle Pine, Minnesota: American Guidance Service, Inc., 1946.

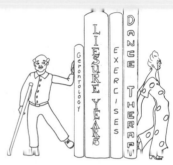

A. Rosenthal

Books

American Alliance for Health, Physical Education and Recreation (ed.) *Dance for physically disabled persons.* Washington, D.C.: American Alliance for Health, Physical Education and Recreation Publications, 1976.

American Alliance for Health, Physical Education and Recreation (ed.) *Dance therapy; focus on dance VII.* Washington, D.C.: American Alliance for Health, Physical Education and Recreation Publications, 1974.

Bernstein, P. *Theory and methods in dance/movement therapy: a manual for therapists, students and educators.* Dubuque, Iowa: Kendall Hunt, 1972.

Birchenall, J. *Care of the older adult.* New York: Lippincott, 1973.

Birren, J. E. *The psychology of aging.* Englewood, New Jersey: Prentice-Hall, 1964.

Braley, W., Konick, G. & Leedy, C. *Daily sensorimotor training activities.* Freeport, New York: Educational Activities, 1968.

Bright, R. *Music in geriatric care.* New York: St. Martin's Press, 1972.

Brunner, D. & Jokl, E. (eds.) *Physical activity and aging,* Kreitler, H. & Kreitler, S. "Movement and aging." Baltimore, Maryland: University Park Press, 1970.

Burnside, I. M. (ed.) *Nursing and the aged.* New York. McGraw-Hill, 1976. P. 255–269.

Burr, H. T. (ed.) *Psychological functioning of older people.* Springfield, Illinois: Charles C. Thomas (3rd ed.), 1971.

Butler, R. N. *Why survive?* New York: Harper & Row, 1975.

Butler, R. N. & Lewis, M. *Aging and health.* St. Louis, Missouri: C. V. Mosby Co., 1973.

Canner, N. . . . *And a time to dance.* Boston, Massachusetts: Beacon Press, 1968.

Chaiklin, H. (ed.) *Marian Chace: Her Papers.* Columbia, Maryland: American Dance Therapy Assn., 1977.

Chapman, F. A. *Recreation activities for the handicapped.* New York: Ronald Press Co., 1960.

Covalt, N. K. *Bed exercises for convalescent patients.* Springfield, Illinois: Charles C. Thomas, 1968.

Cowdry, E. V. et al. *The care of the geriatric patient.* St. Louis, Missouri: C. V. Mosby Co., 1971.

Cratty, B. J. *Movement behavior and motor learning.* Philadelphia, Pennsylvania: Lea & Febriger, 1967.

Cumming, E. & Henry, W. E. *Growing old.* New York: Basic Books, Inc., 1961.

Curtin, S. R. *Nobody ever died of old age.* Boston, Massachusetts: Atlantic Monthly Press, 1973.

Davis, J. E. *Clinical applications of recreational therapy.* Springfield, Illinois: Charles C. Thomas, 1952.

De Beauvoir, S. *The coming of age: a study of the aging process.* New York: Putnam, 1972.

Desnick, S. G. *Geriatric contentment.* Springfield, Illinois: Charles C. Thomas, 1971.

Dunbar, F. *Emotions and body changes.* New York: Columbia University Press, 1954.

Falconer, M. W. *Aging patients: a guide for their care.* New York: Springer Publishing Co., 1976.

Feldenkrais, M. *Body and mature behavior.* New York: International Universities Press, Inc., 1949.

Felstein, I. *Living to be a hundred.* New York: Hippocrene Books, 1973.

Fisher, S. & Cleveland, S. *Body image and personality.* Princeton, New Jersey: D. Van Nostrand Co., Inc., 1958.

Phinney, G. A. *Creative rhythmic movement: boys and girls dancing.* Englewood, New Jersey: Prentice-Hall, 1959. P. 242-243.

Posse, N. *[...]* [...] [...]. [...] Boston [...].

Posse, N. [...] [...] [...] [...] New York: Lyceum Gymnasium, Inc., 1975. P. 181, 182, 183, 184.

Prinzmetal, I. H. *Handbook of geriatrics.* Rossman, I. & Oster, S. W. "The geriatric patient." New York: The MacMillan Co., 1968.

Rusk, H. *The principles of physical care and rehabilitation for patients in nursing homes.* St. Louis, Missouri: Warren H. Green, 1968.

Grabowski, S. & Mason, W. D. (eds.) *Learning for aging.* Hickson, H. A. "Education for physical fitness in the later years." Washington,

D.C.: Adult Association of the United States, 19. P. 250-267.

Harris, J. A., Pittman, A. & Waller, M. *Dance awhile.* Minneapolis, Minnesota: Burgess Publishing Co. (4th ed.), 1978.

Harris, R., Frankel, L. J. & Harris, S. (eds.) *Guide to fitness after fifty,* New York: Plenum Publishing Co., 1977.

Hayes, E. R. *An introduction to the teaching of dance.* New York: Ronald Press Co., 1964.

H'Doubler, M. A. *Dance: a creative art experience.* New York: Appleton - Century - Crofts, 1940.

Hirschberg, G. G. *Rehabilitation: a manual for the care of the disabled and elderly.* New York: Lippincott (2nd ed.), 1976.

Hirschberg, G. G., Lewis, L. & Vaughan, P. *Rehabilitation.* Philadelphia, Pennsylvania: J. G. Lippincott (2nd ed.), 1976.

Homburger, F. *Medical care and rehabilitation of the aged and chronically ill.* Boston, Massachusetts: Little, Brown & Co. (3rd ed.), 1974.

Hornbecker, A. & Frankel, L. *Preventive care, easy exercise against aging.* New York: Drake Publishing Co., 1976.

Illinois State Department of Public Health. *Training manual for a rehabilitation program in a nursing home and an extended care facility.* Springfield, Illinois: Rehabilitation Educational Services, 1967.

Kastenbaum, R. (ed.) *Contributions to the psychobiological aspects of aging.* New York: Springer Publishing Co., 1965.

Kastenbaum, R. (ed.) *New thoughts on old age.* New York: Springer Publishing Co., 1964.

King, F. & Herzig, W. M.D. *Golden age exercises.* New York: Crown Publishers, Inc., 1965.

Klein, W. E., LeShaw, E. & Furman, S. *Promoting mental health of older people through group methods: a practical guide.* New York: Mental Health Materials Center, 1965.

Knopf, O. M.D. *Successful aging.* New York: Viking Press, 1975.

Kraus, H. *Principles and practice of therapeutic exercises.* Springfield, Illinois: Charles C. Thomas (4th ed.), 1963.

Kraus, R. *Therapeutic Recreation Service.* Philadelphia, Pennsylvania: W. B. Saunders Co., (2nd ed.), 1078.

Kubie, S. H. & Landau, G. *Group work with the aged.* New York: International Universities Press, Inc., 1969.

Laban, R. *The mastery of movement.* London, England: MacDonald & Evans, Ltd. (3rd ed.), 1971.

Lefco, H. *Dance therapy: narrative case histories of therapy sessions with 6 patients.* Chicago, Illinois: Nelson Hall, 1973.

Lipson, G. *Rejuvenation through yoga.* New York: Pyramid Books (8th ed.), 1972.

Long, J. M. *Caring for and caring about elderly people.* Philadelphia, Pennsylvania: J. B. Lippincott, 1974.

Lowen, A. *Depression and the body.* New York: Penguin Books, 1972.

Merrill, T. *Activities for the aged and infirm: a handbook for the untrained worker.* Springfield, Illinois: Charles C. Thomas (5th ed.), 1977.

Merritt, M. *Dance therapy programs for nursing homes.* Boston, Massachusetts: Unitarian Universalist Association (revised ed.), 1971.

Mosey, A. C. *Activities therapy.* New York: Raven Press Publishers, 1973.

Pesso, A. *Experience in action, a psychomotor psychology.* New York: New York University Press, 1972.

Pesso, A. *Movement in psychotherapy: psychomotor techniques and training.* New York: New York University Press, 1969.

Pitt, B. M. D. *Psychogeriatrics.* London, England: Churchill-Livingstone, 1974.

Rathbone, J. L. *Relaxation.* Philadelphia, Pennsylvania: Lea & Febriger (revised ed.), 1960.

Reichard, S., Livson, F. & Petersen, P. G. *Aging and personality.* New York: John Wiley & Sons, Inc., 1962.

Rosen, E. *Dance in psychotherapy.* New York: Dance Horizons Republication, 1974.

Rosenberg, M. *Sixty-plus and fit again.* New York: M. Evans & Co., 1977.

Rudd, J. L. & Margolin, R. J. (eds.) *Maintenance therapy for the geriatric patient.* Springfield, Illinois: Charles C. Thomas, 1968.

Salkin, J. *Body ego technique.* Springfield, Illinois: Charles C. Thomas, 1973.

Schilder, P. *The image and appearance of the human body.* London: England: Routledge & Kegan Paul, 1925.

Smith, B. K. *Aging in America.* Boston, Massachusetts: Beacon Press, 1973. P. 196–198.

Spolin, V. *Improvisations for the theatre.* Chicago, Illinois: Northwestern University Press, 1963.

United States Department of Health, Education and Welfare. *Working with older people: Vol. 3, The aging person: needs and services.* Rockville, Maryland: Public Health Service Division of Health Care Service, 1970.

United States Department of Public Health, Public Health Nursing Section *Elementary rehabilitation nursing care.* Washington, D.C.: United States Department of Health, Education and Welfare Public Health Service Publication No. 1436, 1966 (reprint 1970).

Wethered, A. G. *Movement and drama in therapy.* Boston, Massachusetts: Plays, Inc., 1973.

Wolff, K. *The emotional rehabilitation of the geriatric patient.* Springfield, Illinois: Charles C. Thomas, 1970.

Williams, M. & Worthington, C. *Therapeutic exercise.* Philadelphia, Pennsylvania: W. B. Saunders, 1972.

Winter, R. *Ageless aging.* New York: Crown Publishers, Inc., 1973.

Pamphlets

American Hospital Association (ed.) *Winds of change; a report of a conference on activity programs in long term care institutions.* Chicago, Illinois: American Hospital Association, 1971.

Bureau of Special Continuing Education (ed.) *Training for new trends in clubs and centers for older persons; proceedings of a seminar, T.N.T. No. 3 of Ithaca College.* Albany, New York: New York State Education Department, 1968. P. 38–41.

Central Bureau of Jewish Aged (ed.) *The significance of the group activity for the institutionalized aged.* New York: Central Bureau of Jewish Aged, 1970. P. 28, 29.

Hill, K. *Dance for physically disabled persons.* Washington, D.C.: American Alliance for Health, Physical Education and Recreation Publication No. 245–25916, 1976.

Hunt, V. *Movement behavior: A model for action.* Quest, Spring 1964, Monograph No. II, Columbus, Ohio: Ohio State University School of Physical Education, P. 69–91.

Irwin, K. *Dance as a prevention of, therapy for, and recreation from the crisis of old age: A.D.T.A. Monograph No. 2,* Columbia, Maryland: American Dance Therapy Association, 1972, P. 151–190.

Martin, W. C. (ed.) *Aging and total health.* St. Petersburg, Florida: Eckerd College Gerontology Center. 1976.

Mason, K. C. (ed.) *Dance therapy: focus on dance VII,* Washington, D.C.: American Alliance for Health, Physical Education and Recreation Publication No. 243–25570, 1974.

President's Council on Physical Fitness and Sports and The Administration on Aging (ed.) *The fitness challenge in the later years.* Washington, D.C.: Administration on Aging Publication No. (OHD) 75–20802. Reprinted 1975.

Samuels, A. *Dance therapy for the aged: A.D.T.A. proceedings of the third annual conference.* Columbia, Maryland: American Dance Therapy Association, 1967, P. 85–87.

Schwartz, C. G. *Rehabilitation of mental hospital patients: public health monograph No. 17,* Washington, D.C.: U.S. Department of Health, Education and Welfare, 1953.

Thompson, M. *Starting a recreation program in institutions for the ill or handicapped aged.* New York: National Recreation Association, 1960.

U.S. Administration on Aging (ed.) *Facts about older Americans.* Washington, D.C.: Dept. of Health, Education and Welfare Publication No. OHD 75–20006, 1975.

U.S. Public Health Service, Chronic Disease Program (ed.) *Strike back at stroke.* Washington, D.C.: U.S. Dept. of Health, Education and Welfare, (distributed by The American Heart Association) 1975.

U.S. Public Health Service, Chronic Disease Program (ed.) *Up and around.* Washington, D.C.: U.S. Dept. of Health, Education and Welfare (distributed by The American Heart Association) 1974.

Journals

Andrews, G. Preventive geriatrics: is it possible? *Journal of Geriatrics,* November 1970, P. 26.

Ball, E. L. The meaning of therapeutic recreation. *Therapeutic Recreation Journal,* Vol. IV, No. 1, 1970.

Berger, L. & Berger, M. A holistic approach to the psychogeriatric patient. *International Journal of Group Psychotherapy,* Vol. 23, 1973, P. 432–444.

Humphrey, F. Therapeutic recreation and the 70's: challenge or progress. *Therapeutic Recreation Journal,* Vol. VII. No. 8, 1970.

Jeffers, F. C. You and the aging in your community. *The Gerontologist,* Vol. 10, 1970, P. 57–59.

Kraus, R. Reality through dance. *Recreation,* November 1952, P. 326–327.

May, S. R. Purposeful mass activity: a provocative experiment with the aged. *Geriatrics,* Vol. 21, October 1966, p. 193–200.

Menks, F. et al. A psychogeriatric activity group in a rural community. *Journal of the Association of Occupational Therapy,* Vol. 31, No. 6, July 1977, P. 376–384.

Meredith-Jones, B. Moving and living elderly people. *Laban Art of Movement Guild Magazine,* England: No. 27, May 1961.

Reichenfeld, H. et al. Evaluating the effect of activity programs on a geriatric ward. *The Gerontologist,* Vol. 13, Summer 1972, P. 305–310.

Sandel, S. L. Integrating dance therapy into treatment. *Hospital and Community Psychiatry, Journal of the American Psychiatric Association,* Vol. 26, No. 7, July 1975, P. 439–440.

Schoenfeld, L. R. The psychomotor approach in the nursing home. *Dance Magazine,* October 1977, p. 82–84. A look at Americans in the year 2000. *U.S. News and World Report,* March 3, 1975.

Weil, J. Special programs for the senile in a home for the aged. *Geriatrics,* Vol. 21, January 1966, P. 197–202.

Adult Leadership (monthly) Adult Education Association of the United States, 810 18 St. N.W., Washington, D.C. 20006

Aging (monthly) Administration on Aging, U.S. Dept. of Health, Education and Welfare, U.S. Printing Office, Washington, D.C. 20402

American Journal of Dance Therapy (semiannual) American Dance Therapy Association, Suite 230, 2000 Century Plaza, Columbia, Maryland 21044

American Journal of Occupational Therapy (monthly) American Occupational Therapy Association, 6000 Executive Blvd., Rockville, Maryland 20852

Current Literature on the Aging (quarterly) National Council on the Aging, 1828 L St. N.W., Washington, D.C. 20036

Directory of Services for the Aging in New York State (annual) N.Y.S. Office for the Aging, 112 State St., Albany, New York 12207

Geriatrics (monthly) Lancet Publications, 4015 W. 65 St., Minneapolis, Minnesota 55434

The Gerontologist (bimonthly) The Gerontological Society, 1 Dupont Circle, Washington, D.C. 20036

International Journal of Aging and Human Development (quarterly) Baywood Publishing Corp., 43 Central Dr., Farmingdale, New York 11735

Journal of American Geriatrics Society (monthly) 10 Columbus Circle, New York, New York 10019

Journal of Gerontological Nursing (bimonthly) C. B. Slack, Inc., 6900 Grove Rd., Thorofare, New Jersey 08086

Journal of Leisurability Leisurability Publications, Box 281, Ottawa, Ontario, Canada KIN 8V2

Modern Maturity (semimonthly) American Association of Retired Persons, 215 Long Beach Blvd., Long Beach, California 90801

Newsletter of the N.Y.S. Office for the Aging (monthly), Empire State Plaza, Albany, New York 12223

Rehabilitation Literature—abstracts and index (monthly), National Easter Seal Society, 2023 W. Ogden Ave., Chicago, Illinois 60612

S.A.G.E. Project News National Association for Humanistic Gerontology, Claremont Office Park, 41 Tunnel Rd., Berkeley, California 94705

Social Work Journal (bimonthly) National Association of Social Workers, Suite 600 1425 H St. N.W., Washington, D.C. 20005

Therapeutic Recreation Journal (quarterly) National Therapeutic Recreation Society, 1601 N. Kent St., Arlington, Virginia 22209

Adult Education Association of the United States 810 18 St. N.W., Washington, D.C. 20006

American Association of Occupational Therapy 6000 Executive Blvd., Rockville, Maryland, 20852

American Association of Retired Persons 215 Long Beach Blvd., Long Beach, California 90801

American Dance Guild, Inc. 1619 Broadway, Suite 603, New York, New York 10019

American Dance Therapy Association, Inc. 2000 Century Plaza, Suite 230, Columbia, Maryland 21044

American Nursing Home Association 1025 Connecticut Ave., N.W., Washington, D.C. 20036

American Society of Allied Health Professionals Suite 300, Dupont Circle N.W., Washington, D.C. 20036

Ethel Percy Andrus Gerontology Center, University of California, Los Angeles, California 90007

Committee on Research in Dance c/o New York University School of Education, Washington Square, New York, New York 10003

Gerontological Society 1 Dupont Circle, Washington, D.C. 20036

Laban Art of Movement Center, Woburn Hill, Addlestone, Surrey KT15 2QD, England

National Association for Human Development 1750 Pennsylvania Ave.,
N.W., Washington, D.C. 20006

National Association of Social Workers Suite 600, 1425 H St. N.W.,
Washington D.C. 20005

National Therapeutic Recreation Society 1601 North Kent St., Arlington, Virginia 22209

National Council on the Aging 1828 L St., N.W., Washington, D.C.
20036

National Dance Association of American Alliance for Health, Physical
Education and Recreation 1201 16 St. N.W., Washington, D.C.
20036

New England Council of Creative Therapies 20 Rip Road, Hanover,
New Hampshire 03755

Many years of experience on the academic faculties of Brown and Rutgers Universities and the State University of New York have contributed to *Erna Caplow Lindner*'s skills as a workshop leader and writer on geriatric dance therapy. She has earned an excellent reputation training students for educational and therapeutic careers. At present, Erna is an Associate Professor of Health, Physical Education, and Recreation at Nassau Community College on Long Island. She is director and choreographer of a performing dance-theatre company. Her background includes extensive work in creative dance for all ages at educational and community service institutions. Professor Lindner is a frequent member of panels on the therapeutic use of dance. She has given successful courses and presentations for professional organizations such as the American Assn of Sex Educators, Counselors, and Therapists, the American Art Therapy Assn, the American Alliance for Health, Physical Educa-

tion, and Recreation, the American Dance Guild, and the
Zeman Institute for Instruction of the Jewish Home and
Hospital for the Aged. In recognition of her achievements
in the fields of education and dance, she has been cited in
Who's Who of American Women. The activities described
in this book are heavily drawn from her field experiences.

Leah Harpaz draws upon her vast experience as an out-
standing creative dance teacher for children and adults to
develop new approaches for the aging. She conducts many
successful programs in day centers, nursing homes, and
hospitals such as the Jewish Institute for Geriatric Care,
New Hyde Park, New York. The participants in Ms. Harpaz's senior citizen groups at Temple Israel, Great Neck,
have performed for community celebrations. Her background includes extensive training and performing with
leading personalities in ballet, folk, and modern dance. She
is gifted with the ability to communicate with a wide range
of geriatric groups because of her varied cultural experiences and her linguistic talents. She has demonstrated her
unique approaches to geriatrics for members of the therapeutic section of the New York State Recreation and Park
Society. Leah has given workshops on dance therapy at
educational conferences such as at Hofstra University. Her
current community and professional contributions include
service as Executive Vice-President for Dance and movement therapist for special populations at the North Shore
Community Art Center in Great Neck, New York and Co-
Chairman of the Queens Chapter of the American Dance
Guild. The activities described in this book are heavily
drawn from her field experiences.

A leader in the field of geriatric dance therapy, *Sonya
Samberg* has done extensive work in geriatric facilities at
hospitals, rehabilitation centers, old age and nursing

Adult at Hostos, Bronx Community and Queensboro Community Colleges. She has distinguished herself by having introduced dance classes for children into Alaskan public schools. Students in the fields of gerontology and therapeutic recreation studying at Hunter and Lehman Colleges and N.Y.U. observe her workshops regularly. Sonya also conducts therapeutic dance programs for the blind and severely handicapped. Her work shows the influence of a wide variety of movement approaches. She has studied and performed in Modern, Ethnic, Folk Dance and Jazz. She has studied and applied Yoga, Contrology principles of movement, and Sensory Awareness in her work with people of all ages. The activities described in this book are heavily drawn from her field experiences.